MW01383454

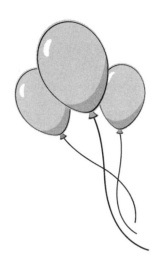

Losing Weight
By Letting Go

You're Carrying Around Stress, Not Fat!

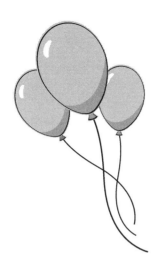

Losing Weight
By Letting Go

You're Carrying Around Stress, Not Fat!

Karen Batenic

Cover Design: Rich Bogucki, Denver, Colorado
Interior Design: The Printed Page, Phoenix, Arizona
Printing by: The Maple-Vail Book Manufacturing Group, York, PA
Photograph of the author by: Natalie Golden, Zoë McKenzie Photography, Chicago, IL
Creative Advisor: Rich Wolfe, Author, Marketer and President, Lone Wolfe Press

First Hardcover Edition: 2009
Hainsworth Associates, Scottsdale, AZ

ISBN: 978-0-9825488-0-6
Library of Congress Control Number: 2009936064

Printed in the United States of America

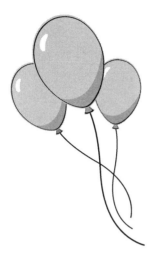

Visit our website: **www.losingweightbylettinggo.com to:**

1. Order a copy of this book to be shipped to you or to someone you think it can help.
2. Send an e-mail note to the author at **losingweightbylettinggo@yahoo.com**
3. Request the author to speak at your group event.
4. Send us a note describing the stress in your life and how it caused you to gain weight.
5. Join our e-mail club

This book is available at a special discounted price when purchased in bulk quantity for group presentations, sales promotions, fund raising or charitable causes.

For details, write a note to:
losingweightbylettinggo@yahoo.com

Karen Batenic is a supporter of the Arts, the Humane Society, and a number of other charities that support women, children, animals, and health issues.

A portion of the proceeds from each book sold will be donated to various charities.

Acknowledgments

It takes the influence of many people to bring an idea to life. I believe that all of the different people that come in to our life have dropped by for a purpose, not just by chance. Everyone we meet has an influence on us in one way or another.

I would like acknowledge and give a special thank you to Jackie, a friend I met by chance through business. We had planned to meet for 30 minutes but our meeting ended up lasting three hours.

Jackie and I found that we were both deep, spiritual people and I was struggling with my purpose. Jackie later sent me the book, A *Purpose Driven Life*, by Rick Warren, which I thoroughly enjoyed. This book gave me the insight and drive to write my success story of weight loss in this book, *Losing Weight by Letting Go*, to help others rid themselves of unnecessary stress and the weight that goes along with it.

My next thank you goes to the three most important people in my life, my daughters. Your love, laughter and encouragement keep me going every day and your belief in me and my ideas kept me moving forward.

Last, a special thank you to John, who introduced me to Rich, who took the time to mentor me and guide me through the world of writing.

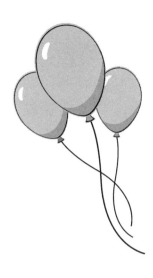

Contents

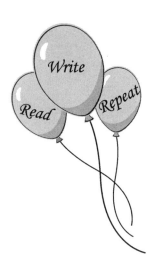

Instructions: Read, Write, Repeat

The key to gaining the maximum amount of help from this book is to take your time and read it slowly. Stop and think about each chapter before you move on to the next. Write down your thoughts and your feelings, no matter how uncomfortable those thoughts might be, or how they make you feel. Then, list the people or situations that cause stress in your life.

You need to write down your thoughts and feelings, as well as your action plans, directly in this book so it becomes your personal journal. This exercise, when complete, will assist you in finally letting go of your stress, and letting go of the people who cause the stress in your life. Every time you are faced with a stressful situation, re-read this book and remind yourself to let go!

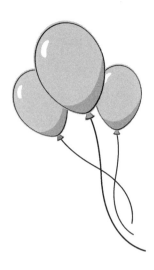

Introduction

Lose Dozens of Pounds Without Exercising!

Marriage – 5 lbs., Divorce – 5 lbs., Family – 5 lbs., Conflict at Work – 5 lbs., Relationships and Break Ups – 5 lbs., Job Loss – 5 lbs. Financial Worries/Debt – 5 lbs., Ex Spouse/Custody Issues – 5 lbs., Raising Teenagers – an extra 5 lbs., Retirement Account Losses – 5 lbs., Medical/Health Issues – 5 lbs. How many of these situations apply to you? As I've found, it's no wonder we're overweight. We're carrying around stress, not fat! That's why I'll show you how to lose weight without exercising.

Losing Weight by Letting Go is a true story and personal journey of how to lose weight by letting go of stress, past hurts, endless worry, and the anger stored deep inside which triggers stress-related eating.

This book is a step-by-step guide which will help you take an excursion deep into your own thoughts, stuffed and buried inside of your inner closet. Through a self-journal, you will learn how to identify, attack, and free yourself of the emotional baggage in your life and the weight gains that go along with it.

Whether your stressor is a parent, sibling, spouse, ex-spouse, lover, ex-lover, child, neighbor, friend, boss, work associate or all of the above, this book is for you. You will be guided through a defined process to identify the stressor, offer suggestions on how to eliminate the stress and/or stressors from your life, and help you lose weight and improve your health in the process.

Once you learn the steps to conquer eating due to stress, you'll watch the pounds melt off, and stay off, without even exercising!

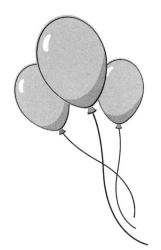

Chapter 1

It's All About Stress

*H*ow many times have you tried to lose weight, or committed to start a diet on Monday, (or maybe it was every Monday)?

Maybe you just wished that you could wake up one morning at a comfortable or "perfect" weight and maintain it from there? Those were the thoughts that I had on a regular basis until I found that successful weight loss truly wasn't about a diet, but about managing the level of stress in my life.

My own weight was weighing me down both emotionally and physically. Once I discovered the secret of *Losing Weight by Letting Go*, I was ready to get off that weight see-saw so many of us are stuck on, and start taking back control of my life!

Personally, I have lost dozens of pounds in a total of four months, **WITHOUT EXERCISING**. Plus, I have managed to keep this weight off for over two years now. I was able to drop the pounds, and keep them off, by letting go of anger, past hurts, and all of the stress and stress related eating that was associated with those pounds.

I had been carrying around the weight of those extra pounds that I wanted to lose for the past 14 years.

First, I blamed the excess weight on my thyroid. My metabolism must be slowing with age I thought, but the doctor said that wasn't the problem.

I then tried all of the fad diets that made the headlines. Through the years I tried the grapefruit diet, the cabbage soup diet, the Atkins Diet, the South Beach Diet and Weight Watchers many times over. Most of those diets were tolerable except for the Cabbage Soup diet. For all of you who have been continuous dieters, you might have tried that crazy plan. You would basically starve yourself all day and then your evening reward was cabbage soup. I didn't like cabbage to begin with, so even though I was extremely hungry, cabbage soup hardly felt like a reward. When I nearly passed out from a lack of calories, I gave up on that diet. There would always be another Monday to start something new.

The latest fad diet that I had been hearing people talk about was the "cleansing diet". This diet is very unhealthy as you are expected to consume only water mixed with syrup, and cayenne pepper. What a weird combination! It just goes to show how desperate people are to lose weight. They will try anything and are willing to risk their health just to lose some weight quickly. These fad diets usually never last, and the weight that is lost usually returns very quickly.

For long-term successful weight loss, there is a right way and a wrong way to lose those unwanted pounds. The wrong way, such as starving yourself or consuming too few calories, will only result in a return of the temporary weight loss with feelings of failure when the weight returns. A strenuous workout regime will work temporarily but will not keep the pounds off long term unless you keep up this same work out plan for the rest of your life.

The right way to lose weight is the healthiest and easiest to maintain over time. It consists of eliminating stress from your life and making wise food choices. **Plus, when a person is mentally ready to lose weight, they will lose it successfully.**

All of the best rewards that we receive take some time and effort; it's the same for long lasting, successful weight loss.

Through the years of my experimentation with fad diets and simultaneously carrying around my extra pounds, I always managed to include some sort of exercise in my life. I had been power walking twice a week, for an hour and a half, consistently for the past ten years, even if the weather was nasty.

Power walking was an enjoyable activity for me; to walk and talk with my friends, but it never seemed to help me lose much weight. It kept me energized and toned, but it didn't get me to my desired weight or back into that old pair of jeans from college.

With each diet that I tried, about 5 or 6 pounds would come off fairly quickly, but the weight would always seem to reappear much faster than it ever would ever disappear. My "baby" was now 18, so using childbirth as an excuse for my extra weight was no longer an acceptable reason for me even though I convinced myself for years that that was the problem. It was time for my baby weight to go away and stay away.

Embrace our Differences

People come in many different shapes, sizes, and colors. We may be tall, average, or short in height, we may have any variety of hair color, we may have curly hair, straight hair, or no hair. We have different eye color, and we all come in a multiple of sizes which can vary through the years. Our closets usually hold a variety of sizes and at least one pair of jeans from a point in time where we were at our lowest weight; hoping to fit in them again some day.

We are unique individuals and we all have our own comfort zone with weight. Although I was comfortable with my appearance (as long as I wore black and kept out of the eye of the camera), I knew this wasn't the real me. Pictures were deceiving, I thought. No one photographs well, would echo through my mind when I would see a picture that was not very flattering.

We've also been told over and over again that the camera adds ten pounds, so that would be another excuse that I would think of when an unflattering picture of me would present itself. Or maybe I just happened to be bloated that day, I would convince myself... Whenever photographed, I became the master of hiding half of me behind someone else in a picture, or finding a spot to stand in the back of the group to be sure that there was a short person in front of me.

Sometimes when being photographed, I would try to remember what Oprah said the correct pose was to get the slimmest angle from the camera and then try to maneuver into that pose before the camera clicked and froze that image in time.

The real me was 30 pounds lighter, wore bright colors, enjoyed being photographed, ate a variety of foods, and didn't gain weight. I didn't understand how the first 25 years of my life I did just that and remained thin!

I knew that metabolism slowed with age, but there had to a better explanation as to why my body now maintained this comfort zone of extra weight, primarily in the mid-section, right below the breasts and above the belly button.

Since the diets weren't working, it was time to find out why I wasn't losing weight. To do this, I had to spend some alone time with just me to figure out what caused my hunger, my constant consumption, and my weight gain. I knew I wasn't eating enormous portions, but I had to admit "nibbler" could have been my middle name and I was "nibbling" more than I ever wanted to acknowledge.

Acknowledging my weakness was a very difficult step for me to take. I needed to take the time to be alone and just think about me, how I felt and what was on my mind; this was not a comfortable task for me at first. I personally had a habit of always being in motion (this was to avoid thinking about what was really bothering me). There were chores to do, work to occupy my time, and with children, no mater how old they were, there was always somewhere to go or some-thing to do that would distract me until I would fall asleep at night from exhaustion.

Once I stopped all of the self-made continuous motion, and devoted time to just me, I was able to take the time to determine when I ate, what I ate, and what triggered my appetite for something to eat quickly. By doing this I was able to shed my extra weight **WITHOUT EVEN EXERCISING!** I'd like to share my success strategy steps with you.

Losing Weight by Letting Go

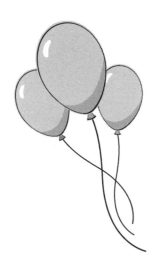

Chapter 2

Alone Time

Step 1—Alone Time

The first step which I took was to take the time to identify what was going on in my life.

The urge to explore why this extra weight would not go away on its own was overwhelming. I needed to designate a block of time where I could focus on just me and my thoughts.

As difficult as this might be to accomplish, it was time to change my routine and schedule. I needed to carve out at least one hour of time—several days per week—where I could just think about my own life.

I was so busy taking care of everyone else on a daily basis that there was no time left for me.

There were kids to take care of, backpacks to empty, homework to check, endless shopping and cooking, doctor appointments to make, attend, or drive someone to, bills to pay, laundry to do, family to check in on, friends to help out, trying to maintain some sort of a social life, and this all had to be done besides working full time at a job with a two hour commute!

Being a woman made me a caretaker of everyone but myself. This is a role that many women fall into and that is why so many women get angry over time. Women naturally take on the caretaker role and men gladly let them have it! It seems to be a successful plan and this works for a while—then this plan blows up as the silent resentment builds through the years and women then become tired of so much responsibility with so little thanks. And so we eat.

I knew with so much responsibility that it would be difficult to find any time for me but I knew it was something that had to be done, and had to be done quickly. Otherwise, my stress level would continue to increase causing either illness, depression, or even more weight gain.

In order to be able to make some alone time for me, I had to decide what could be put off until the next day so that I would be able to take an hour for myself. This hour had to be either in the morning or early evening because if I waited until everything was done and everyone else was taken care of, I was too tired to think. All I wanted to do by evening was to lie down, put my tired feet up, and go to sleep.

My decision was to put some of the daily chores on hold, such as dishes and laundry. Those two chores never seemed to go away so if I skipped them one day it didn't really matter; there would just have to be a double load to finish the next day. This change in my routine allowed me to set aside one hour, three times a week for some reflection time.

This new found time was a bonus that broke up my usual daily routine. I had to make a promise to myself to not let anyone else steal this time from me. It was time to explore what was "eating me".

On my first hour of alone time, I decided that I would need to start writing down everything that I ate; to make a food journal that would also include my thoughts and feelings. At first, the thought of keeping a food and emotional journal sounded like just another chore for me. However, after reflecting, I realized that it would be helpful to have all of the facts in front of me before I could truly make a determination of what I might be doing wrong in making my food choices. To be truthful and factual, I would need to write down when I would eat, what I would eat, and what drove me to eat.

My new commitment would be that my log would include every bite, chip, sip or spoonful that I put into my mouth.

In the past, when trying to keep a food journal, I would tend to "not count" the one bite here or there consumed when cooking. That was just a taste I would think, too small to bother to write down. I never acknowledged the calories that were in all of those little tastes. I also never seemed to count any food that wouldn't technically hit a plate. If I would grab some delicious, salty cashews right out of the can and pop them directly into my mouth, I never bothered to acknowledge that snack as calories consumed. Or, if I grabbed a few hot, golden, French Fries from someone else's plate or carton, that too would never count as calories consumed. In fact, any food consumed while not sitting down, usually never made it to my food log in the past.

Standing in the pantry while staring at the shelves and looking for something to cook, usually resulted in sneaking a few salty, crunchy chips from a bag (not counted). Or, when

11

opening the fridge to see what was inside, this would usually result in reaching in and taking a bite or two of something in there while I was staring at the contents (not counted).

The cool breeze of an open fridge is mesmerizing for some reason. It's easy to stare inside as the tempting foods whisper "taste me".

Another discovery that I have found while staring into the open fridge, was that leftovers sure taste good when cold, especially pizza! There have been times (usually on a Monday) when I would be all set to start my day with a diet plan of fresh fruit and cottage cheese. The plan would fail when the fridge would open and my eyes went directly to the shelf with the cold pizza wrapped in foil begging me to take a bite. One bite would turn into one piece, then another and another until I was too full to eat the cottage cheese. That would now have to wait until next Monday when a new diet would begin.

Or, another situation that would present itself would be when cooking and stirring something delicious in a warming pot on top of the stove, it would be typical for me to taste what was simmering to see if it was seasoned right or hot enough. When you are hungry and stressed, it's easy to keep sampling. Sometimes those tastes alone could have added up to enough calories for a mini-meal, but they too were never counted. I know I'm not the only cook who does this.

Many dieters I have talked to have acknowledged that they have done the same thing or would underestimate the portion size of food consumed. By not counting every single bite we consume or sneak, or not considering if our portion size is small, medium, or large, or not realizing that every topping we put on a sandwich loads on tons of fat and extra calories, we are only deceiving ourselves. **It's like cheating at the game of solitaire when playing cards!** What is the point?! I was now ready to commit to my food/emotional journal-without cheating. I would be loyal to my log.

Taking Time to Think

After thinking deeply, I found that for me, my hunger was induced and magnified by stress. Without even realizing it, or acknowledging it, I was under a tremendous amount of stress.

I was working full time in a management position, and in addition, I was raising three daughters on my own for the last 14 years. I was maintaining a home, and now several cars as my daughters were now all old enough to drive. I was in the middle of a costly and lengthy court battle with my ex-husband over child support and college expenses. On top of that, a relationship that meant a lot to me had just ended and added sadness to my life.

Through more alone time, I discovered that in order to address my feelings and explore all of the items that were truly causing my stress, I would need to spend several hours on a regular basis in solitude with no distractions from music, TV, or my family.

I needed to finally slow down and face what was causing and adding to all of this stress in my life.

If I kept busy as usual, I could stay distracted from what was really bothering me. I found that talking on the phone, watching TV, listening to music, or surfing the internet would keep me occupied enough to not think about things that were upsetting me or causing me stress. This is because the

13

brain cannot process two distinctly different thoughts at the same time. So rather than taking the time to pause, and think, I just kept busy and ate instead. Those are two things that you can do at the same time!

Somehow the food comforted me, temporarily, and then made me feel horrible about myself later. While an ice cold creamy chocolate milkshake tasted so good at the moment of consumption, at home later on I would become angry at myself for ruining another "diet day."

After thinking about it, it wasn't that I was hungry but the stress in my life caused me to reach out for something com-forting—fattening food or drink. Plus, when mad at myself, my behavior was then to lash out at someone else—who-ever happened to be nearby.

As I would reflect back during my deep thinking periods, I thought that I ate fairly healthy.

I always had breakfast (a double chocolate doughnut and black coffee was my favorite). I would remove the skin off of chicken. I would drink skim milk instead of whole milk. I rarely ate fast food. I hardly ever ate dessert and I would stay away from deep-fried foods.

However, I wasn't noticing that every time I had a rush of stress, whether it was from a bill in the mail, an upsetting or stressful phone call, a letter, a conflict situation at work, or a stressful encounter with someone, or especially a confron-tation with my ex, I would get this panic urge to eat something quickly. That usually included something choco-late as that was always within reach, or to quickly grab some type of bread and lather it with butter. This quick consump-tion seemed to tame my stress for a little while.

After lots of thinking, what I found was that other people can also pass on stress to us even when we are unsuspecting. For example, an angry person in traffic can cut us off, a co-worker might make an insulting remark, a boss might criticize our work unnecessarily, or a spouse or parent might make a comment that will hurt deeply because they know us well enough to hit our vulnerable and insecure spots.

All of these items can cause stress which in turn will cause an immediate reaction for some of us to grab a piece of food, and when we do grab something, it's usually not an apple.

When suddenly hit with a stressful situation or comment, I found that I wanted to eat something really quick. The stress alarm sound would go off in my belly which in turn made my brain focus on food. This put my eyes in motion to seek out a sweet or salty item to basically inhale until the stress urge passed, not realizing that it was the feeling that had just been fed.

When on a food search, what I found that was always readily available in the office, or at home, seemed to be candy, cookies, coffee cake, ice cream, doughnuts or Danish, or some type of a salty snack like potato chips or pretzels.

On my own, (thinking this was a healthy option) I would carry a quick snack fix of some mixed nuts, or a mozzarella cheese stick, in my purse for those sudden hunger snack urges. I really thought the salty nuts and high fat cheese were healthy alternatives instead of eating candy! I had picked up this idea from a previous diet.

Although nuts can be healthy, when under stress, I would eat a large handful or two of cashews, not just one or two nuts, which were very high in fat and covered with salt. At other times, I would eat several pieces of cheese. A few pieces of cheese didn't seem like much food, and I knew mozzarella was a low-fat cheese, but I wasn't considering how much fat and how many calories it was taking to satisfy this stress beast inside of me.

The portions seemed too small to possibly be doing any true weight damage, I thought. These snacks tasted great and my stress seemed to be relieved temporarily after eating them. These high fat/high salt foods did the job and satisfied my stress-related hunger urge, but they did nothing to change or eliminate my stressful situations.

In addition, they seemed to induce my appetite to want even more of the same types of fatty, salty type of foods. The stress, along with the extra pounds, remained very loyal and stayed right by my side.

Now that I identified that I ate quickly accessible, high fat/high sugar or salty, unhealthy snacks when under stress, I decided I had to start eliminating the stress from my life, not just change the way that I ate.

I had tried changing my diet over and over in the past. This approach did not seem to be working for me as I would never stick with my new changed diet for the long term. In fact, I would tend to "mix" diets.

I might start off the day counting points but if I had a large portion of meat, I would decide to be on a high protein diet by the end of the day. The next day I would start fresh with another type of diet until I walked into the office and someone was celebrating some event—with doughnuts or a layered whipped cream cake of course!

For some reason it is really hard for me to pass up a dough-nut-especially a Dunkin' Donuts Double Chocolate one. They are my favorite and as soon as I see one that Dunkin' Donuts jingle pops into my head—"It's time to make the doughnuts" and my hand grabs the delicious treat before the brain can say no. All of this mixing of diets did not work so I would consciously decide to eat whatever I wanted for the rest of the week and vow to start fresh the next Monday.

The Monday fresh start approach had been drilled into my mind from long ago, I think from my mother, with the myth that you can eat and drink whatever you want on the week-end if you follow a regimented diet during the week. This is not true and does not work!

There is no need to diet to lose weight. The key to weight loss is through managing stress. This time, my approach would be to eliminate the stressors which caused me to grab a quick fix of fat and sugar—if I could—and see if that would make a difference in my life, and in my weight.

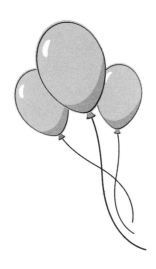

Chapter 3

Reflecting

Step 2 — Making a List of Stressors

To continue on my journey of self-exploration, I managed to keep putting the chores on hold and kept my designated commitment of one hour, three times a week held for me to ponder my stress and its effect on me.

I needed to take the time to think all by myself in a quiet setting. I found this was very difficult to do; to just focus, identify, and think about the key stressors in my life.

Avoidance is a much easier path to take rather than to address a conflicting or stressful issue or person.

Most people do not want to jump into conflict and address it head on, but this needs to be done in order to eliminate the stressor permanently from your life. If you try to just bury the stress, it will keep popping up from its hiding place at inopportune times and the conflict or stressor will never be resolved.

For example, if there is someone in your life that you have a past conflict with, until you address the conflict and confront the real issue the two of you have, you will constantly feel that sense of apprehension when they are around. It is that stressful feeling you have when you feel your jaw tighten and a slight flush will creep through you from your head to your toes. Your brain tells you that you want to verbally attack this person but you condition yourself to hold back and keep your feelings buried deep inside.

Other comments that might be said, which are unrelated to the conflict, might cause you to feel anxious or stressed when you are around that person. However, it all returns back full circle to the original point of conflict. Until that particular conflict item is addressed and resolved, you will continue to bury this conflict inside causing more stress, pain or weight gain and possibly sickness to yourself.

I noticed this stress/conflict condition between two of my daughters. For years, they managed to throw out insulting or snide comments to each other at every opportunity.

I knew that kids fought but they were no longer teenagers and were now young adults. I thought that if we do not resolve this issue soon, they might carry this grudge on in to the future and lose out on having a close relationship as adults; and I didn't want this to happen.

Deep down my two daughters loved each other and would do anything for the other if needed, but the jabs and insults were getting to be too frequent. Besides, this friction only occurred between these two sisters while neither of them ever insulted their younger sister. Since this seemed to be a behavior that happened specifically between these two girls, as a parent I needed to step in and get them to address and resolve the issues that were causing their conflict.

I finally took each one to the side and asked that they think about what was the real problem/conflict that they had with each other. They were told to think about this issue and not give me an answer immediately.

When did this conflict start and what caused the conflict that had been going on for so long between them?

Each one came back to me and shared a hurtful comment the other had made years and years ago, when they were in their early teens. I said that I would not break their confidence and tell the other one, but that they needed to sit down with each other, when they were ready, to hit the conflict head on. They would need to tell each other what the comment was, how badly it hurt, and how that was what was still really causing their conflict today.

It took a few days, but the girls did sit down and I played the role of the referee. They each opened up about the hurtful comments made from years back that were said to each other in a rage of anger.

The Scenario

As a teenager, my daughter Kay was a bit shy. She was a top student in grammar school and high school, and participated in lots of activities and sports. She had nice friends but never got involved with the party crowd. My other daughter Elle, had struggled a little in grammar school and through her first year of high school. Her grades were not the best since she did not make studying her top priority, but she was very outgoing and had numerous friends over to our house all of the time.

People were naturally attracted to Elle. So, having two daughters close in age, living in the same house and going to the same school, but mixing in two totally different crowds, resulted in lots of conflict. They would fight over small items like a borrowed pony tail holder, a shirt one had worn without asking the other for permission, who would get to use the car that night, etc. but the big conflict came of course over a misunderstanding about a boy and war was declared in our house.

Assumptions and anger that was never addressed caused them to throw insults at each other repeatedly throughout the years. These hurtful words and comments, made so many years ago, which touched on each others insecurities and vulnerabilities, caused them to fight like cats for years to come.

When they finally sat down and discussed the cause of their conflict, and took the time to listen to each others side of the story, both girls were surprised by how petty and silly their interpretation of the situation was.

The girls could barely remember the name of the boy that caused all of this fury and they each then had the opportunity to explain their side of the story and the reason they were trying to hurt each other years ago.

The girls had their discussion but they did not hug and say it was all ok when they finished talking. However, they did say that they were sorry, that they never realized the words they used in the past had hurt that much, and that they would be respectful enough to never use those words again since they now knew what tender spots they were for each other.

Now that they shared their vulnerability, I can only hope they will respect each other enough to know that those past remarks are off limits in future fights and if they ever have a major conflict again, they need to take the time to address it with each other rather than make assumptions and hold in their anger.

We cannot minimize the effect name calling has on us when we're kids. Name calling, labeling, teasing, and bullying truly hurt and stay with us affecting our life and our weight until we learn how to **Let Go**.

All About Bill

I came across an example of this recently as I ran into a boy that I went to grammar school with.

Bill was now a grown man and I hadn't seen him in over 40 years. Our grammar school had been large and there were about 100 kids in each grade. We spent those formative years of Kindergarten through eighth grade together.

We lived in a fairly poor inner city area of Chicago, a primarily Catholic neighborhood where the area would be referenced by the name of the parish or church nearby. It was a neighborhood where the frame and brick houses were mostly two-flats and they were so very close to each other that you could look out of your bedroom window and right into the kitchen window of the house next door.

Most families living in the neighborhood included somewhere between three to six kids living in each house. There would always be a baseball game going on in the street as the kids on the block would gather together after dinner. We were a very tight group and most of us knew the brothers and sisters in everybody's family as they would be only a grade or two apart from us.

Very few people ever relocated to another neighborhood, yet alone another state back then, so the whole group of kids grew up together very tightly.

When I finally arranged to meet Bill and his wife for our scheduled dinner, we laughed and commented how we both looked good and hadn't "aged" at all.

Within one hour of our dinner conversation he brought up how he remembered that in grammar school I had been placed in the "smart" room and he spent his time in the "dumb" room.

We had been in school together 40 years ago. When he made that comment the memories of the classroom labeling came right back to me as well. How sad, I thought, that after all of these years that the mean comment and labeling that some-one in our class threw out remained with him. He was a handsome, successful man with a beautiful wife but the label was still buried deep inside of him.

After dinner that night, as I was starting to think about my own issues from the past, I realized that I was becoming more comfortable with taking the alone time I needed just for me. I was now starting to treasure my solitude periods, time which I would have never thought that I could find for myself but now had, now that I just prioritized differently. Chores and errands could wait.

For the first time in my life, I was going to make the time for me before anything else.

Making a List

During my alone time, I would ponder and think. My next step would be to then sit down and make a list of the things that were causing me stress. I'll call these my stressors, which I kept in a notebook that I carried with me everywhere that I went. I wrote these stressors down in this small note-book so that I could be reminded every day of what was causing my stress.

I viewed the stressors as the enemy, and I would keep the enemy close to me in this new journal to help monitor its effect on me and to change its control over me.

Writing down stressors is a way to help the mind peel away layers of hurt and anger.

Just as we used a diary when we were young to write down our precious thoughts and feelings, the journal today would be for identifying and letting go of past hurts, anger, and feeling of unfairness.

By writing these stressors down, I would now be the one in charge, and would eliminate this stress to my body, which in turn made me snack or eat without even realizing it. It was time for the power to shift over to me.

Everyone has their own stress list and we all stress out over different things. Some people can handle enormous amounts of stress and others cannot deal with small amounts of stress. There is no correct measurement for stress as it is unique for each person, but stress is real and it can be damaging.

Through a routine check-up, my doctor informed me that my sugar levels were getting a little too high. Since I rarely ate dessert (remember, chocolate doughnuts are a breakfast food) and I didn't have a "sweet tooth", the sugar levels from my blood work took me by surprise. After looking into the issue, I found that too much bread or pasta can increase sugar levels. Plus too high of sugar levels can lead to diabetes. I certainly didn't want to damage my health over stress related eating since I now knew that this was the reason for my extra pounds and my poor food choices.

To give you an example of what was bothering me, I'll share with you my own personal stressors.

My stress list consisted of the following six major items:

- The latest three-year court battle I was having with my ex-husband over child support and college expenses for our three daughters. We were in court when we got divorced. We were in court again six years later over child support, and here we were another six years later back in court again for the same reasons.

This time we both had busy lawyers that were stretching the issues out as well as a judge that kept canceling and changing our hearing dates. Between their three schedules constantly changing and issues getting postponed, this battle kept dragging on.

Every time we showed up in court it put me behind financially even if there was nothing resolved; just a new date put on the docket.

From this latest battle, there was so much anger that I was holding in as well as feelings of unfairness which had built up to exploding levels in me.

Over the years we were divorced, my ex-husband chose to not assist me in the daily tasks of raising our daughters.

When we first divorced he told me that he would never take the kids for a weekend so that I would never have any free time for myself. That is the one promise to me that he did keep.

While he was able to sleep late on the weekends and have a full social life as he pleased, all of the homework, scheduling, sports, chauffeuring, doctor appointments, and discipline was completely left to me to handle along with working a full-time job; there was no weekend for a single mom.

He would see the girls on select holidays that he picked for a few hours, and he managed to free himself from all of the daily responsibilities that went along with having a family.

The responsibility as well as the expenses would all fall to me.

The job of raising children with two parents is a very difficult task, but single parents have an enormous job filled with responsibility and endless hours of work, and little, if any, time left for themselves.

What I didn't realize, as I fought this battle over support, was that all of the stress associated with this fight was damaging me both mentally and physically. Plus, the total of the legal fees that we both spent on attorneys could have paid for one child alone to go to college. Instead, we both wasted that money by arguing via the lawyers.

The lawyers were just doing their job, but each one was counseling us, telling us we could win this fight which just caused it to be dragged on way too long.

We were divorced—the marriage was over—we should have both stopped fighting over money and addressed what our real conflict was. We didn't, and the legal bills kept piling up.

While all of this **stress with the ex** was going on, I was managing to hold down a full-time job.

- At the same time, a co-worker who reported to me, that I had trusted and totally supported, was back-stabbing me at every opportunity throughout the entire organization.

This behavior took me by surprise as I am a very loyal manager and have always done my best to stand by anyone who works for me and do my best to guide and develop them.

I had much success in mentoring my employees in the past, and would often get notes and cards from those who I developed that moved on to higher, more successful opportunities in other companies. I had mentored both men and women of varying ages, men and women of different races, and men and women at different levels in their career.

Never before had I been faced with someone that I was guiding, supporting and developing, who would be so devious and hurtful behind my back, talking negatively about me and tearing down all that I was working on.

What was most disturbing was that Carol was very nice to my face, almost to an extreme, and was constantly bringing me cards and little gifts.

There was always a card and a balloon for boss' day, my birthday, or other random holidays. This card and gift giving made me uncomfortable as the department head as I didn't want anyone to think that these items could influence me or my judgment. In addition, I think these actions made it uncomfortable for the other people that worked for me.

I didn't want, or expect, cards or gifts at work.

Plus, I didn't want anyone else to feel obligated to do this just because Carol, who reported directly to me, was doing that.

I just wanted everyone to do their job, and to do it well.

Thinking about the situation, I noticed that I was becoming a little bit suspicious of Carol's behavior. However, I dismissed my thoughts and considered that maybe it was just her style or maybe it was the way things were done at this new company that I had just joined. I knew every business had its own culture and maybe the company culture at this location was just different from other company's that I had worked for.

A few months went by and Carol started to share comments about her peers to me. She was telling me who came in late, who took long lunches, who did their school work on work time, etc. As I listened, I tried to determine was she being extremely loyal to me or was she being a gossip.

Since our relationship was still new and she was my direct report, plus she was so professional in her dress and demeanor, I chose to trust her without having her earn my trust. I was hearing about so much of the bad behavior that was going on with the rest of my staff that I really appreciated having Carol's input.

Several months later, a few managers who I worked with closely and had found truly trustworthy, came to me and told me about the negative comments and remarks that Carol was making about me.

Jack overheard Carol speaking extremely negative about me as he was doing construction work in her office area. She didn't even notice that Jack was working right there as he could overhear her comments as she carelessly talked negatively about me, her manager. He genuinely wanted to give me a "heads up" to help me in my new position.

Mike, a manager that I also worked closely with and found trustworthy, came to me and told me how Carol would tear me down in meetings she had with peers when I wasn't present. I listened to both Jack and Mike as they told me this information, never commenting and never sharing to the other what I had already heard.

Since these instances of backstabbing were coming to me from two independent sources, and from successful managers in the organization, I knew they had to be true. Neither Jack nor Mike, who were informing me of these comments, had anything to gain from sharing what they overheard. They were my peers and were truly trying to let me know what was happening in my own department.

The disappointment that I felt was overwhelming. When an enemy attacks, you expect that action. **When someone you trust attacks, the hurt is more devastating.**

From that point on, I started to lose the trust in Carol that I had initially given. I then began my own investigation of Carol's behavior. This was a new company that I was now working in and I was starting to wonder just who could really be trusted.

After effectively digging through information and interviewing others, I found out more about the situation.

To my face, Carol tried to give the impression that she was the only one in the group who worked hard and was a loyal employee. Behind my back, Carol attacked me personally and professionally to anyone who would listen

Since she had been at the company for five years prior to my arrival, she knew many people in the business so there was always an ear for her remarks.

Since I was the new person who was in charge, she had a willing audience as others wanted to hear what she had to say about me, and from there, judge me.

However, as time went on and I established my own relationships, Carol's so called trusted friends were repeating to me everything she said about me word for word.

During my continued investigation, I found that back-stabbing was a pattern for her and something that I should not take personally. It still was hurtful though, and I learned a valuable lesson from it.

It turned out that the rest of the staff was doing their job; they might have been a few minutes late by stopping for coffee, but all of Carol's gossip was exaggerated. Carol was just making things up about them so she would stand out and look better than the rest.

Through my years of listening and coaching in business, I found that it was often that people would repeat their behavior, whatever it was, in a consistent manner. It could be consistently good or consistently bad, but it would usually be consistent. Keep that in mind when selecting friends, a date, a spouse, or a staff member. **Past behavior is usually an indication of future behavior.**

■ My next stressor was that my daughter Elle, who was in college, was arrested for having a false ID. Elle was succumbing to peer pressure with too much drinking while she was living on her own, out of state, away at college.

31

I remember when I was a student in college, everyone had a fake ID, but today the ramifications are much more severe with the focus on terrorism, and also with the appropriately severe punishments for driving under the influence.

A false identification is taken very seriously and you can be arrested, go to jail, and/or pay large fines. Our under age students need to be aware of this so they don't make a bad choice today that could alter their life forever.

Neither Elle nor I realized how serious of an offense having a fake ID is today until it was too late and she was arrested.

Even now I hear parents laugh and say a fake ID is not a big deal, that everyone has one, just like they had in college. Most people still don't know how serious of a crime it is now considered; things have changed.

Next, as an involved parent, I was also concerned because Elle (the middle child) was planning her first trip out of the country with friends. To add to the stress, she would be in Dublin for St. Patrick's Day! Plus she was still under the age of 21. It was bad enough having her in another state pushing the independence envelope to the max, but to think of her being in another country kept **my stress level at a continuous high**.

As a single parent I didn't have anyone to discuss these concerns with and she didn't have a participating father who would give her some words of wisdom, direction, or guidance; it was just me nagging about something else.

I thought of everything that could possibly happen or go wrong — and then I grabbed some candy, chocolate with lots of nuts and chewy caramel of course, to ease my stress. Not just one piece, but multiple pieces from the box which tasted so good at the time and was so soothing to my stress.

As a parent I knew that I had to let Elle learn from her own mistakes, but I loved her so much that I couldn't just let her make bad choices without giving continued input as a parent; even though she really didn't want to hear anymore from me. She was at the age of trying to be independent and thought she had all of the answers and that nothing could hurt her. And so, I ate.

- Next, as I jumped back into the stress of my work day, I discovered that I was feeling some extra job stress as I was the only female on the team in the company that I worked for. Even though I had faced this quite a bit during most of my career, in the highly male industry I was now in, I felt excluded on a daily basis and was not comfortable knowing that the rules were not being applied to me the same way as they were to the men. So, I nibbled to fill the void and the lack of inclusion I felt at work.

As a woman in the workforce for many years, I had often been the only female in meetings throughout my career. While working in a corporate setting, I had experienced a little bit of exclusion, but not much to mention, and all of my interactions with the men I had worked with had been extremely professional.

There were the random occasions where a man, usually married, would hit on me at a meeting or while out of town, but once I relayed that I was there to work and not play, he would return right back to professional behavior and that would be the end of it. However, when I took a role in an operations environment, everything was different. I felt like I had stepped back in time. Now being the only female on this team which included six men and me, was uncomfortable just because I was a woman.

I could handle the inappropriate jokes, the male bonding after hours as they networked playing some type of sport together, even their runs to the bikini bar, but what I couldn't understand was when we were discussing true business there was a code of commitment a few had, **not all of them**, where if one would disagree with me on a subject the other two would jump in and support their buddy whether it made sense or not, at my expense.

This caused me to feel isolated, deflated, and not willing to speak up and bring my ideas to the table anymore. The more this happened, I turned into an office recluse and drifted away from any interaction with any of the men on the team, even the three who had always been fair to me.

This feeling of exclusion, isolation, and loss of motivation caused me a tremendous amount of stress which in turn caused me to complain to my friends, family, and significant other and **to eat—endlessly**.

Looking back, I should have stopped putting so much energy into complaining and put that same energy into something constructive to remedy the situation.

When I finally took the time to explore this stressor in depth, I found that I was **expecting exclusion** from this all male team and so some of my own actions caused the exclusion to happen.

Some of these feelings of exclusion were a reaction to my actions which I wasn't aware of until I finally came to realize it during my alone time.

However, just like any situation, a portion of this discomfort was due to my expecting exclusion but a portion of how I was treated was also because it is still hard for some men, not all, to accept a woman in a leadership role. While the majority of the men I worked with were considerate and fair, there were a few that had their own ideas and issues about women who made it incredibly difficult for me to work with.

- Also during my alone time, I came upon and faced the realization that I was soon to be an empty nester. My baby, nicknamed Gooey, was now 18 years old, and was heading off to college in the fall.

This would be the first time in 24 years that I wouldn't have any kids to care for at home anymore.

After being a parent for the last 24 years, my youngest child was now ready to leave home and go off to college. I was excited for this event, but I was also apprehensive about the loss and no longer being needed as a mom.

All of my hurried schedules, attending multiple sporting events, and juggling three kids and a full time job would soon be over.

The fear of the unknown was overwhelming to me and the thought of being alone was frightening and stressful.

The more I thought about it, I knew the anxiety was also a feeling of where had my life gone? Did I accomplish all that I wanted to do or was I just rushing around taking care of everyone else? I wasn't even sure what it was that I wanted to accomplish — I had been too busy working and raising kids to even give that any thought.

The years had flown by and I was so used to putting myself last that I wasn't sure what I would now do with my time.

Many women that I have talked to have expressed that they too have felt this feeling of loss when their children leave for college. It is the same feeling of loss that women feel whether they have been working moms or stay at home moms. All of a sudden you notice your age, your mortality, and that you are now making room for the next generation to achieve and experience all of the things that you have already gone through.

When a child leaves, it is a huge adjustment to the home and feelings of emptiness are constant. However, the good news is that we adjust in time. All of a sudden there is a freedom to do whatever we want and to be able to focus on ourselves, but I didn't know this at the time.

- My final stressor, which I had identified on my list, was that I had been dating a man for over a year who I felt was kind and generous and very loving. I was very happy and fulfilled when I was with him. He made me laugh constantly which helped to release some of my stress.

He pursued me intensely with cards, flowers, and calls when I wasn't sure that I even wanted or had time for a serious relationship. Then, after months went by and when I finally let my guard down and let him totally become a part of my life, we broke up.

It happened so fast that I didn't see it coming. After devoting over a year to him and spending all of our free time together, there was now an immediate emptiness in my life when he just packed up and left and moved to a different city. I felt this hurt deeply now on top of all of the other things that were adding stress to my life. Later I wondered if this was just his pattern.

I had now figured out that when stressed, I ate. And, since I was under a lot of stress, I ate a lot!

I will call this action to a reaction a food trigger.

Next, I determined what it was that I ate under stress. It turned out to be high fat/high sugar foods or salty, quickly accessible foods, such as chocolate, nuts, cheese sticks, coffeecake, doughnuts, bread with butter, or some type of salty bag snack like chips or pretzels.

All of these items were easily accessible in an office or home setting, and took no cooking time. These things all tasted so good to me at the time. So, when I wanted something quick, or when a surge of stress came over me, one of these items would be readily available and quickly do the trick and fill the void and loneliness in my life.

Time for Things to Change

I had made up my mind that things were going to change and it was time to declare war on my weight and stress.

To do this, I took each stressor I had identified and broke it down into components. I did this to form each stress-related item in my life into a set of manageable steps to attack and permanently eliminate from my life.

This would now become my official **WAR ON WEIGHT.**

Each stress item on my list seemed on its own to be over-whelming to me with no solution in sight. However, as I thought about the stress related items and I outlined several steps to remedy each one, each stress-related issue seemed like it could be resolved and eliminated from my life.

By attacking the stress and breaking it down into several **small steps** to attack and eliminate it, it no longer seemed like an impossible task to remove from my life.

Each person has their own level of tolerance for stress. Some people can handle a lot of stress while others crumble under minimal stress.

As we are each unique individuals, no one should feel bad if what is stressing them out might not stress out another person. Stress is a true condition that we need to eliminate, whatever the level might be to you personally. Stress affects our weight and health, our well being, and our relationships with others.

When under stress, we tend to snap or react in a negative way that just passes on the stress and negative feelings to the next person who is available. That person then takes the negativity, which they in turn pass on to someone else and the negativity just keeps on flowing.

Think of how you might start a day in a really good mood and then all it takes is one snide comment or a negative attitude from someone to turn your day around and make it unpleasant and stressful. It's time for that to stop. We need to practice passing on good thoughts and good comments to others so that is the energy force that is dominant.

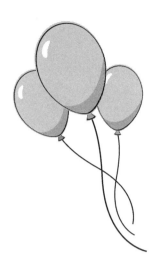

Chapter 4

Sharing

*W*hile on my journey of *Losing Weight by Letting Go*, I attended a Divorce Recovery workshop at the community church near my house, which is called Willow Creek.

I had been raised Catholic but had been disappointed that the Catholic Church never offered any assistance to divorced people, only to widows. Although I can't even imagine the pain a widow might feel, the death of a marriage through divorce is also very painful, damaging, and more common. Yet our traditional churches do not seem to address the loss and pain associated with divorce. Although Willow Creek was not my regular church, something drew me to search their website to look into this program even though I was well over my divorce. I had healed years ago from the cheating and his betrayal and now I was just angry that I didn't receive help from my ex.

I had attended a few Sunday services at Willow Creek throughout the years and found their approach to life problems through the study of the Bible was very interesting and reflective. An old friend of mine had gone to Willow Creek for divorce recovery years ago and I remembered that they offered some type of program.

My divorce had been over for 14 years now, even though my ex-husband and I were still fighting over money and support issues.

I researched, and then attended, the Divorce Recovery Workshop originally as I was so distraught over the recent relationship breakup that I had just gone through. This break up had felt like another divorce to me. After spending two weeks in the program, this Divorce Recovery program helped me to see that it was years of stress, hurt, and conflict in the earlier years of my life that I was continuously grieving over, not necessarily this particular relationship that had just ended.

By participating in the Divorce Recovery group program and sharing with other men and women, who were also letting go of hurtful feelings or relationship loss, we formed a bond of understanding.

I can't even remember the last names of the people in my group, but we shared our hurts and pain with each other in a safe, non-judgmental forum. Hearing the tremendous pain others had gone through gave me the ability to be grateful for what I did have, learn to accept everyone for who they were, work on changing myself not others, stop complaining about issues current and past, and start making the changes to alter any situation that I was personally unhappy with.

We have more power in our own thoughts and actions than I ever believed possible. I then linked the two together that the stress I continuously felt is what in turn caused me to eat.

I spent a total of 24 weeks in the Divorce Recovery program, continuing to sign up for three sessions of eight weeks each, which I recommend to anyone who has experienced any pain or relationship loss in their life.

Any relationship loss can be shared in this confidential group setting. You do not have to have been married to attend a Divorce Recovery session. Relationship breakups hurt deeply and we need to help others heal who are hurting. The program at Willow Creek helped me to focus and then **let go**. In addition, because of the program's healing techniques, it also reinforced my belief that with God at my side, I was never alone. With God for me, who could be against me? These were powerful forces that were now with me at all times.

Recovery Sessions

During the 24 weeks of Divorce Recovery sessions, I found that I had so much bottled up inside of me that I wanted to say. The three hour sessions which were held once per week, flew by each evening that we met as a group. Years and years of injustices, long past verbal abuse that I had been subjected to, and negative experiences that occurred during my marriage flowed out of me and were shared with my group members. Issues from long ago that I had buried deep inside of me were now coming out to strangers. Once I was able to speak of it, it was then released from my body and I was then able to heal.

Each week I couldn't wait to meet with my confidential recovery group. No matter how tired I was or what the weather was like, I would attend the session. When the first eight weeks were finished I knew I had to continue as this program was helping me so much. As the weeks went by, from one to 24, I kept speaking but found what I had to say was lessening each week. At my 24th week, I finally ran out of things to say and I was able to attend and just listen as new members would share their pain.

I finally understood how the leaders could just sit there all night and listen; it turns out that they had all been participants themselves at one time or another and were now giving back and helping others by facilitating these sessions. As the new people joined us, they had their opportunity to unload the things that had been hurting them for years and the healing process continued. We were finding that past hurts from early in a persons life affected not only their self-esteem but the way we would seek and handle relationships later in life. We found that it was necessary to heal properly first, before you could ever truly move on to the next relationship if you wanted that next relationship to be successful.

If you didn't heal, it was likely that you would just continue to repeat the previous pattern of behavior that was in the last relationship.

I never would have thought in meeting with a group of strangers that I would open up and share some of the most hurtful events and comments that I experienced in my life. However, as the others shared, we saw we were not alone in this healing effort and that the support from others, both men and women, was incredible.

The number of weeks each person needs to heal is an individual decision. For me, 24 weeks is what I needed to feel free from the hurts. Others left the group after the first 8 weeks and some had completed a full year of sessions. No one pressures you to continue. It is a voluntary program that is designed to help others heal and the counselors are marvelous people who give back to others what they have learned via the Bible.

Horrible, insulting words from a loved one whether it is a parent, spouse, lover, sibling, or child, can be devastating and have a lasting impact on us.

Negative, hurtful words can shatter a person's self confidence and cause many to feel worthless. I found others in my group, both men and women, who had been the victims of a cheating relationship who were devastated and broken from it. The women seemed to be able to speak of their hurts immediately while most of the men just sat there and listened. After several weeks of listening, the men then began to share their hurtful stories. I think they needed to feel safe in the environment before they were able to share. Some of the men would show up for several weeks and then disappear for several weeks. When they would finally decide to return they felt safe enough to speak. It was a touching experience to hear how both men and women had the same hurts and issues to share.

However, the most heartbreaking stories to hear were from those who were physically abused. You cannot imagine the pain and suffering, both physical and mentally, that some people have gone through. Physical abuse occurs in all ages, races, sex, and income levels. No one should ever allow another person to hit them or to deflate their self esteem through insults and name calling.

Hearing other people's stories helps to put your own hurts into perspective. Just when you think your situation was really bad, you find someone else who has experienced things much worse.

This is a step in the healing process where you can start to feel grateful for all of the things you do have, all of the people you have loved, and all of the people who have loved you. When you hear about how much silent suffering is going on it helps you to **stop being judgmental of others**. You never know what is happening behind closed doors in someone's life so we need to make an effort to be kind to other people and look for the good rather than the negative.

After hearing about all of the hurts that people have been exposed to, from family members or from someone they were in a relationship with, you can sympathize with them or show empathy, but the greatest gift is to just listen and not comment. Listen to others express their pain. As they express it, it is then released, and it is gone.

The key is to listen in a non-judgmental manner and not offer solutions. Just having someone listen allows those who have been storing hurts the ability to let some of the hurt go.

When someone has physical pain, they are able to scream to release some of their pain. When someone has emotional pain they need to do the same in order to release it from their body rather than just hold this pain inside. This can be in the form of talking, writing or just screaming about the hurt/pain felt until it is released from the body.

Holding in emotional pain can cause distress or illness to a person. Men are often told to "handle it", to not show their feelings or to bury their emotions deep inside. However, if you bury the hurt it will never heal. If you don't heal, your next relationship will probably fail and the **cycle will not change until you change;** not to mention the toll it will take on your body and the weight you will gain from the stress.

Emotional hurt will cause you to lose your self esteem and self worth. While some people deaden their pain with alcohol and/or drugs, others will try to do the same thing with food.

We will work on changing this so that we will eat when hungry, not when stressed.

We will work on moderation with alcohol to enjoy it as it is intended and not use it to numb feelings.

Drugs are a means of self-destruction. If you can't enjoy yourself without drugs, you are missing out on life and all that it has to offer, and should seek professional help for your hurts and emotional pain.

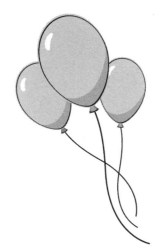

Chapter 5

A Personal Action Plan

Weekly Steps to Lose Weight by Letting Go

A Personal Action Plan...Ready, Set, Go!

Week 1

The first thing you will do this week to start your *Losing Weight by Letting Go* program, is to acknowledge your stress.

What stresses out one person, may not stress out another person. Some people can handle incredible amounts of stress and others fold at minimal amounts. Remember that you are a unique individual and no one else can feel how you do, and that is completely acceptable! Accept this, and how you feel, and realize that just talking about your stressful situation or gaining sympathy from friends and/or family will not resolve it. *You*, and only you, need to take action to remove this stressor from your life.

You can do it. **You will be successful**, and you will be determined to make the right changes in your life.

Your first step to begin this journey of weight loss is to spend some time alone, in silence, either sitting outdoors, or spending time at a park, or by taking a walk all by yourself.

If you think that there is no time for you to devote to yourself, you need to make time. Get up a half an hour earlier or go to bed a half an hour later, put off any chores for a day if you need to, but be sure to make the time just for you. Try to not have any distractions during this precious alone time. You shouldn't have a friend with you, or children, or even a pet. This time is just for you and your thoughts so that you will not be distracted and can concentrate on what is causing your stress.

Next, think deeply about what or who is causing your stress. After you've thought this through, **write down what or who causes the stress in your life**. Be honest, this will be your confidential log. Even if you start to feel guilty if the first person who pops into your mind that adds stress to your life happens to be a spouse or relative, write it down. There are no wrong answers, these are your feelings!

After you have identified who adds stress to your life, then write down as many as six stressful situations that you are involved in.

You might have more stressful situations than that, but six is a manageable number to begin with. After the first six that come to mind are conquered, you can move on to the next six. The stressful situations could be due to a person (spouse or lover, an ex, a sibling, a child, a friend, a parent, a step-parent, a work associate, boss, or neighbor), a remark someone made to you (a current remark or a remark made in the past, or ongoing jabs and insults), or just how someone treats you in general. Does someone belittle you, make you feel sad, inferior, not intelligent, unattractive, fat, worthless, strip you of your confidence, or make you mad or angry at the way they treat you? If yes, list that person.

By writing down who this person is will be your first step of letting go. It will be your way of acknowledging who is causing your stress and how you will no longer let this person dump this stress upon you which causes you to eat in excess. A stressor could also be an event, finances, or an addiction. List each one down individually after you've thought about it deeply. We are going to conquer these stressors. Think about who, what, when, where and how they make you feel.

Week 1: Personal Worksheet

Keep this worksheet in a private place so that you may write down your thoughts and comments freely and honestly.

List the People or Situations That Bring Stress Into Your Life:
1.
2.
3.
4.
5.
6.

You have made the first step towards Losing Weight by Letting Go.

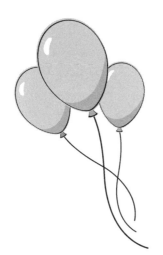

Chapter 6

Cleaning Out Your Cabinets

Week 2

Now that you've made your list of who, or what, is causing your stress, you will need to review this list every day. Keep your list in your pocket, purse or wallet, or in a notebook that you carry with you at all times. Note your feelings when you look at your stress list and especially note if those feelings make you want to eat something to make the pain or stress go away.

During Week 2, while evaluating your stressors, you will need to help rid your body of excess sugar to curb the stress cravings. Make these food changes/swaps in your life for the next two weeks. You can do anything you put your mind to for two weeks when you choose to do so. Remember that these food replacements are for the next two weeks, not forever. If you cheat, you are only cheating yourself and stopping the process of Letting Go.

Review the following list of foods and drinks to eliminate from your life for the next two weeks. **ELIMINATE THEM**

FROM YOUR HOME and eliminate them from what you order in a restaurant. Do not leave an open bag of chips, pretzels, or cookies in your house. When you keep that product in sight, sooner or later, one by one those chips and crackers will disappear and before you know it the bag is empty.

If you keep a bowl with candy in your home or on your desk at work, you will need to get rid of those as well. Avoid these temptations and be prepared with the replacement foods listed below when you are ready to start your two weeks of healthy body cleansing.

In addition, by not keeping any of the foods listed on the elimination list in your house, when you are faced with a stressful situation or feel the need for a late night snack, there will not be any poor food choices available for you. If it is not there, you cannot eat it. Again, this is only for two weeks until you can see how you will lose your taste for these foods naturally.

Eliminate	Replace With
Regular Soda	Diet Soda or Water
Whole Milk	Skim Milk/Fat Free Milk
Half and Half	Skim Milk
Glass of Juice	Glass of Water or Club Soda with a splash of juice
Sweetened Tea	Unsweetened Tea (do not add any type of sugar substitute)
Waffles, Pancakes, Bagel, Toast, Muffin or Doughnut	One Egg cooked any way you like
Omelet	Egg Beaters mixed with any fresh vegetables
Cheese	Fresh tomatoes
Nuts (any type)	Non-sugar coated cereal

Eliminate	Replace With
Sugar Coated Cereals	Oatmeal, Special K, Corn Flakes, or Rice Krispies
Bacon	Canadian bacon or a Ham slice
Cream Soups	Broth-based soup (You can also put a broth based soup like minestrone into the blender and liquefy. This will give the appearance and texture of a cream soup but without the cream and the fat and calories associated with it.)
Chicken with Skin	Chicken with Skin Removed
Lunchmeat (Beef & Pork)	Only sliced chicken or turkey lunchmeat
Pork Ribs	Grilled pork chop only
Pork sausage	Chicken, turkey, or vegetable sausage only
Beef	**Lean** ground beef or steak only, nothing processed
Sandwich	Salad
Salad Dressing	Soy sauce, Balsamic Vinaigrette, or BBQ sauce, fat-free salad dressing or fresh squeezed lemon juice (Always on the side, not tossed in the salad)
Bread, Hamburger and Hot Dog Buns	Substitute lettuce for bread and buns for the first two weeks, then switch to low calorie whole wheat bread. Look for the bread that has a calorie count of less than 50 calories per slice. (Suggestions: Healthy Life Brand, Weight Watchers Brand or Sara Lee Delightful Brand Bread)

Eliminate	Replace With
Rice, Potatoes, or French Fries	Fresh steamed or stir-fry vegetables (no sauce added)
Pasta with any type of sauce	Whole wheat pasta, not regular, with marinara sauce only
Pizza	Homemade meatballs with marinara sauce
Tacos	Taco Salad (no sour cream, no tortilla bowl)
Salty Snacks/Bagged Chips/ Pretzels	Fresh fruit or low-fat yogurt or sugar free applesauce
Any dessert including cookies, ice cream, and cake	Jell-O fat free/sugar free pudding (any flavor) with a dollop of whipped cream. Be sure to mix the instant pudding with skim milk for a delicious dessert. OR Fresh fruit OR A banana topped with Smuckers fat-free caramel sauce (heat the sauce in the microwave) and topped with a dollop of whipped cream OR A banana with peanut butter smeared on one side and then topped with Honey Bunch of Oats Cereal. This is a fantastic, satisfying, healthy dessert.

Eliminate	Replace With
	OR Fat free yogurt with fresh fruit added and cereal topping. OR Fat free yogurt with fresh fruit added and cereal topping. OR Slice an apple and sprinkle ground cinnamon on top and two tablespoons of Smuckers fat free caramel topping and bake at 350 degrees for 30 minutes.
Butter or Margarine	Olive oil or vegetable oil spray
Mayonnaise	Mustard or ketchup
Sauces	Lemon juice or bbq sauce
Croutons	Eliminate from your salad
Frozen Foods	Replace with a fresh item
Canned Food	Replace with a fresh item (exception soup)
*Salt	Pepper

*Salt may cause you to retain water and carry excess water weight. It may also raise blood pressure in some individuals. Using salt may be a habit that you have; try to eliminate using salt and you will see that you will hardly miss it after two weeks.

This is not a diet. This is a lifestyle change for the way you will eat.

You should notice that by starting your day off with a protein item, an egg for example, you will not be as hungry as you would normally be if you started your day off with a sweet or bread type of item. When you eat something sweet, the body continues to crave more sugar and it is likely that you will eat more bread, pasta, and desserts than you would if you would have started your day with some protein.

The following items are what I call food accessories—clear them out of your house for the next two weeks. If they are not in your house you will not be tempted to eat these items:

- ❏ Any type of nuts
- ❏ Candy
- ❏ Cookies
- ❏ Cupcakes
- ❏ Muffins
- ❏ Doughnuts
- ❏ Pancakes
- ❏ Pie
- ❏ Cake
- ❏ Ice Cream
- ❏ Cheese
- ❏ Mayonnaise or Miracle Whip
- ❏ Tartar Sauce
- ❏ Or Like Products
- ❏ Sugar Substitute
- ❏ Sour Cream
- ❏ Syrup
- ❏ Potato Chips,
- ❏ Tortilla Chips
- ❏ Pretzels

- ❏ Popcorn
- ❏ Any Bagged Snack
- ❏ Crackers
- ❏ Bread, Garlic Bread, and Rolls
- ❏ Buns
- ❏ English Muffins
- ❏ Tortillas
- ❏ Creamy Salad Dressings
- ❏ Rice
- ❏ Potatoes
- ❏ Regular Pop/Soda or Sweetened Drinks

All of these items are accessories, not necessary for your meals for the next two weeks. You will be able to have full meals without any of these items.

By eliminating these items from your diet for awhile, you will lose the urge to snack. It's similar to getting dressed without wearing jewelry. You can still look nice, just not accessorized.

After you've completed this process, go
to the grocery store and stock up on
the items listed below. This will
become your shopping list for the
next two weeks!

- ❏ All types of fresh fruit
    - ❏ Apples
    - ❏ Bananas
    - ❏ Plums
    - ❏ Red or Green Seedless Grapes
    - ❏ Oranges
    - ❏ Watermelon
    - ❏ Raspberries
    - ❏ Pineapple
    - ❏ Cantaloupe
    - ❏ Honey Dew Melon
    - ❏ Pears
    - ❏ Strawberries
    - ❏ Blueberries
    - ❏ Raspberries
    - ❏ Peaches and Nectarines
    - ❏ Lemons
    - ❏ Lime
    - ❏ Sugar Free Applesauce
- ❏ Any type of fresh vegetables (except potatoes)
    - ❏ Onions (white, green and red)
    - ❏ Celery
    - ❏ Red and Green Peppers
    - ❏ Green Beans
    - ❏ Broccoli

- ❏ Corn
- ❏ Zucchini
- ❏ Garlic
- ❏ Pea Pods
- ❏ Peas
- ❏ Bean Sprouts
- ❏ Yellow Squash
- ❏ Tomatoes
- ❏ Lettuce And Spinach
- ❏ Cucumber
- ❏ Carrots
- ❏ Fresh Garlic
- ❏ Mushrooms
- ❏ Cauliflower
- ❏ Lean meats such as 93% lean hamburger, steak, and pork chops (preferably all fresh, not frozen)
- ❏ No sausage unless it is chicken, turkey, or vegetable sausage
- ❏ Canadian bacon
- ❏ Chicken (remove the skin or purchase skinless)
- ❏ Turkey or chicken lunchmeat
- ❏ Any type of fish (never breaded or fried)
- ❏ Shellfish
  - ❏ Frozen Shrimp
  - ❏ Crab Legs
- ❏ Eggs and/or egg substitute
- ❏ Peanut butter
- ❏ Low fat/ low calorie yogurt
- ❏ Breadcrumbs
- ❏ Marinara/pasta sauce (jar is fine)
- ❏ Whole wheat pasta

- ❑ Canned soup (non creamy)
- ❑ BBQ Sauce
- ❑ Soy Sauce
- ❑ Salsa
- ❑ Pickles
- ❑ Ketchup
- ❑ Mustard
- ❑ Vegetable spray for cooking
- ❑ Lawry's Sesame Ginger Marinade and other low calorie flavors
- ❑ Coffee
- ❑ Tea (unsweetened)
- ❑ Diet Pop
- ❑ Juice
- ❑ Skim/Fat-free Milk
- ❑ Cereal (non-sugar coated)
- ❑ Quaker Oatmeal
- ❑ Balsamic Vinaigrette Salad Dressing and any other fat free salad dressing
- ❑ Sugar-free, fat-free puddings made with fat free milk
- ❑ Smuckers fat free caramel sauce or hot fudge
- ❑ and a can of whipped cream for a small topping on your pudding or banana.

Now study your stress list and condition yourself to grab a piece of fruit if just reading about the stress items on your list causes you to long for a food trigger/accessory.

You are preparing yourself to Lose Weight by Letting Go.

You will be successful! You will feel better! You will look better!

60

Week 2: Personal Worksheet

Review these tasks and when you have completed each one, initial and date to acknowledge your progress.

TASK	Date	Initials
1. Empty your refrigerator and cabinets of Food Accessories (or move them to a separate drawer that you will not use and that will not be in your immediate sight.)		
2. Rearrange your refrigerator, cabinets, or pantry and keep all of your "replaced foods" in a location of easy access.		
3. Go to the grocery store and purchase only "approved" foods for your next two weeks.		

GREAT JOB!!

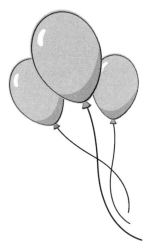

Chapter 7

Attacking the Stressors

Week 3

You are now ready to attack and eliminate the stressors from your life. You have conditioned yourself to grab only a piece of fruit, or sugar-free applesauce, or fat-free sugar-free pudding when you get a stress related hunger urge. Even though it might be tempting to grab some chips or pretzels, you won't because those items are no longer in your house.

Your family can do without these bagged snacks and food accessories as well for two weeks, so do not keep a supply on hand for them. It will be too tempting for you to have these items around when something stressful comes your way during your first two weeks of this process. You will also be helping your family by helping them to change the way they eat as well.

If your family will not assist you while you are attacking your stressors, keep their "stress" foods in a separate cabinet out of your view and ask them to put everything away in its proper hidden location so that you will not be tempted to sample one of these items while under stress. Then, the next time you are spending some alone time thinking, explore why your family will not support you on your Losing Weight by Letting Go journey for two weeks. If your health is not important to them, make sure it is important to you.

When on the go, you should keep two pieces of fruit with you at all times so you are prepared and not tempted to reach into a community candy bowl. These "sugar bowls" are everywhere we go—in the office, at the bank, on the hostess stand in a restaurant, etc. A banana, an apple, or a little bag of grapes all travel well and are easy to keep on hand. In addition, the individual sized containers of sugar free applesauce are easy to keep in your purse, car or at work. Fresh fruit will be less expensive than purchasing individually packaged fruit and fresh fruit will not contain any syrups or preservatives. Get in the habit of bringing home fresh fruit like watermelon and cantaloupe and cutting it up immediately and having it always available for snacking in a bowl in the refrigerator.

Next, start reviewing each of your stressors one at a time and break each down into the following components:

- How have I contributed to this stressful situation? List your role in each stressor. Be honest with yourself here. Even though your role may be small, every action you take creates a reaction so you need to admit what your contribution to this stress situation is or was. If you think that you have not done anything to contribute to this stressful situation, you need to go back and focus more on this stressor and identify what part you had in it, even if it was small. There is always some remark or action that we have taken, not necessarily wrong, that caused the reaction that someone else has given to us.

For example, if you are always nice and friendly but the person you are having a conflict with is rude in return, you need to think if you are latching on to someone who is either verbally abusive, a bully, or who has such low self-esteem that he or she wants to strip you of your self-worth to feel better about themselves.

Note if this is a pattern you have and if you are consistently picking people as friends or lovers who don't treat you as well as you treat them.

YOU need to break this cycle and start searching for good people with the same morals, values, and ethics that you have.

Week 3 Personal Worksheet I

Complete the chart below. You have already identified your stressors. Now add what role you played in each stress situation. Be honest. This is your confidential record to help you Lose Weight and Let Go.

Stressor	Your Role/Action or Words that Contribute to the Stressful Situation
1.	
2.	
3.	
4.	
5.	
6.	

Keep these notes hidden in a safe place so that you are comfortable in writing things down truthfully.

Review the role that you have played in the stressful situations above. Look to find if there is a pattern of conflict situations or if there is a pattern to the contribution you make to these stressful situations. Once you acknowledge your role/contribution, you'll be able to change this behavior in yourself. This doesn't mean that the stress is your fault; it's just that there is usually a pattern to behavior. If you are constantly the giver or the victim, note this particular pattern down. If you constantly "give" but the recipient hurts you in return, you need to think if this behavior might be a pattern from long ago. It might be a role you observed a parent perform so if it's all you know, this negative behavior might "feel like love". Start changing the behavior to get different results or start changing the type of people you select as friends or those you have a relationship with.

Week Three: Personal Worksheet II

Next, you need to think about how and why others have contributed to this stressful situation that you are a part of. List who and what they have done, and why they have contributed to each stressor. Is there something in their own life pattern that causes them to act this way or are they repeating a family hurt/behavior that has been passed on to them?

Remember that you cannot change others, just yourself. So if you are in a relationship that you find yourself saying that he or she would be perfect, if only he or she didn't .... (fill in the blank), then you are deceiving yourself. You cannot change that person so if they are not right for you, either accept that person for who they are or move on.

Find someone or something that does make you happy as is—without having to make any changes.

Stressor	Role of Others and Their Behavior History
1.	
2.	
3.	
4.	
5.	
6.	

Week 3: Personal Worksheet III

As you are continuing your process of deep thinking, ask yourself, is this stressor in my control to fix? Or am I the cause?

- ❏ If yes, the stressor is in your control to fix, fix it by writing down multiple actions/steps that are needed to achieve this goal;

- ❏ If no, if the stressor is not in your control to eliminate, remove yourself from the situation and view the situation as an outsider would. Think about what advice you would give a friend who was in this situation that you are now faced with. Then, list those steps that you would advise someone else to take to eliminate that particular stressor from their life. We can all see things more clearly when it doesn't affect us. Try to give yourself the same advice that you would give a close friend or someone you care for deeply.

Stressor	In My Control to Fix?		Role of Others and Their Behavior History
	Yes	No	
1.			
2.			
3.			
4.			
5.			
6.			

- Next, write those steps down and take that advice yourself one little step at a time without saying "but....". Don't think of all of the reactions that could or might happen by taking these steps, just write down the steps you would advise a friend to take. Try to be as objective as you can with this exercise. As you work through this process and break problems down into tiny steps/components you will find that the results and proper outcome will always be there for you. When life problems are too large and seem over-whelming, this is the perfect way to solve the problem. You will be surprised at how your own thoughts will help you find a meaningful solution when you break the problem down into small steps/components.

Review your list of stressors again to see if there is a pattern that surfaces around what causes your stress. If there is a pattern, start reacting in an **opposite** manner from what your first reaction might be. This will cause a reaction that is different from what you would usually receive. Note/write down the reactions of others when you change your actions/behavior. If this change in your reaction/behavior produces positive results, make the change permanent in how you react.

Your next step will be to focus on the stressors (1 - 6) and **select the one that is the least difficult to eliminate** from your life. Once you have completely thought through the issue, write down your plan of elimination.

This plan might include taking a break for a while from a person who causes you stress (even if it is a relative or spouse), or finding a new job if the job is causing you too much stress. If one of your stressors is job related, that is usually an easy stressor to correct. There are so many jobs out there you will always be able to find a different one, even in a down economy.

Trying something new even temporarily might open up a whole new career path that you had never even thought of before and when you are in a new job you will always meet new people who might end up opening up new doors or friendships for you.

A job is not a marriage so it's not intended to be a commitment for life. Try new jobs to see what you like to do and what you don't like to do. You'll meet lots of interesting people along the way and this will add to your total life experience. A change in a job can be the start of a whole new adventure for you. You need to be true to yourself.

If you are bored in your job, or your boss or the culture is trying to alter you into someone that you are not, it is time to move on.

We are amazing, unique, individuals. There is not one correct way to think or perform. We need to embrace the differences we all bring to an environment, so if you're not being appreciated or acknowledged, find some place where you will be. Don't let yourself get into a rut of not enjoying your life and watching the years go by. Do what you like — as long as it is legal and it doesn't hurt anyone else.

When you explore your thoughts when reviewing your stress list, and if you find your stress is due to an improper work environment, be aware that there are many internal opportunities for you to report and correct this improper work situation. Some steps to correct an improper work situation would be to call the anonymous company hot line to report any wrong doing. Most major companies have a toll free number that employees are urged to call if there is something inappropriate happening in the company. This number is usually posted on bulletin boards near employee break areas. You are able to call in anonymously and report your thoughts or findings. These calls are anonymous and will not be traced back to you. The management of the company then has to conduct an investigation into the issue.

Another opportunity for resolving workplace issues is by meeting with the company head of human resources or the legal department. These people are there to help you. Or, if you are not comfortable with any of these options and do not want the conflict in your life, take the time to find another job. It's your choice and you need to take the steps to resolve the issue that work best for you.

Once your action plan is outlined and you start to take the steps you have written to eliminate this stressor from your life, you will then be able to **"Let Go"** and you have just lightened your internal load. By starting with the easiest stressor to eliminate, you will be able to see that there is a remedy, as every problem has a solution. It's the law of mathematics.

One achievement will motivate you to repeat this successful process and remove that stress from your life. Once you accomplish this you will see how your appetite and craving for high calorie/high fat food has changed.

Repeat this with the next stressor and the next until all six are resolved. Once you have mentally accepted that you are working to let the issues go, you will **lose the weight** that was associated with that stressor **permanently.**

From my own personal experience, I have found that each stressor in my life accounted for approximately five pounds of excess weight. After I resolved to eliminate one stressor from my life, and followed my steps of cleaning out my cabinets, I broke my stressor down and completed my outlined steps. When successful in eliminating that stressor, I lost five pounds. As I resolved another stressor and chose to let go, I lost another five pounds. This continued as I lost 25 pounds and lost my appetite for any food accessories.

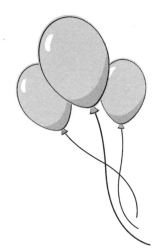

Chapter 8

You're Ready to Let Go!

Week 4

Your list of stressors should now be complete and your breakdown of components /steps to attack these stressors should be completed for each one. You cannot resolve a stressor until you accept that a part of each conflict is due to a contribution that you are making as well as the other person.

Even though your contribution may be small, it is there. Think about what you do, how you say things, or how you act that might cause a reaction in some people. If the reaction is positive, you are doing something right. If the reaction is negative, review your words, tone, style or actions to see how you might deliver the same message if you were to do it over.

Next, select the easiest stressor to resolve and tackle it head on. Enter notes into your chart every day as you tackle each stressor until it's resolved. Work on one stressor at a time to keep focused rather than moving from one stressor to the other. You will need to focus all of your attention on the one stressor until it is resolved, finished, and removed from you life so that you can lose the weight by letting go.

Week 4: Personal Worksheet

Stressor #1

Issue/Person _____

Date	Action Steps to Eliminate the Stressor

Week 4: Personal Worksheet

Stressor #2

Issue/Person _____

Date	Action Steps to Eliminate the Stressor

Week 4: Personal Worksheet

Stressor #3

Issue/Person _____

Date	Action Steps to Eliminate the Stressor

Week 4r: Personal Worksheet

Stressor #4

Issue/Person _____

Date	Action Steps to Eliminate the Stressor

Week 4: Personal Worksheet

Stressor #5

Issue/Person _____

Date	Action Steps to Eliminate the Stressor

Week 4: Personal Worksheet

Stressor #6

Issue/Person _____

Date	Action Steps to Eliminate the Stressor

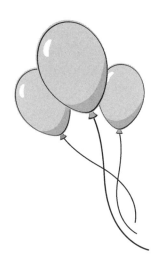

Chapter 9

My Personal Experience of Letting Go

*W*hen I completely reviewed my list of stressors, my final decision was that the first stressor to address was #4; the feelings of discomfort in my office setting.

I needed to think deeply about what caused the discomfort that I felt and why I was extremely stressed in this job. I started to list all of the things that came to my mind when I focused just on that.

I wrote down my thoughts (components) on my log very quickly as they would pop into my mind, not allowing me to first filter these thoughts. First reactions are the best and are usually the most accurate as they are not filtered by our own conditioning and values. My breakdown of components for this stressor was as follows:

I was the only female in a leadership team of six. There were five men and me. I realized that the make-up of the group was not going to change. I had to either accept the situation as it was, or move on to a more diverse business environment. It is very difficult being the only female on an all male team. The jokes are different, the pre-meeting chatter is different, and I would never be a part of the after work socialization and bonding.

The guys were able to get together after work for a drink or golf together on the weekends, but if a divorced female would join them, the other wives would get mad or rumors would start to spin hurting my credibility. So, the men were able to create a bond outside of work that I would never be able to be a part of. Group dinners were fine and inclusive and everybody participated in those; but it was the after dinner activities where I didn't fit in and could not bond as the others did, nor did I want to. For example, the after dinner trips to the strip club or the late night bar.

Even early on in my career I had experienced being one of only a few women on the work team but this was the first time that I was the **only** female.

My first step in attacking this stressor was to make a list of all of the issues that I perceived to be unfair or where favoritism had been extended to several of the men I was working with. They were buddies and when deadlines weren't met or projects failed there were no repercussions for them due to this outside bond. I noticed that the women throughout the organization, including me, were held to a much higher standard. After compiling a list of actual situations that I was sure of, not a list of emotions or gossip, I made an appointment with my boss to discuss my notes. This list was now a fact sheet which was thorough, factual, and lacked emotion as I thought it through in my alone time.

I kept a list of instances I would reference during our discussion to keep me focused and factual. I was prepared, which was very important when making mention of issues of unfairness that had occurred in the workplace.

I decided that the right method to address the problem was with the person who could help resolve it. I would no longer be whining and complaining about this to my lover, friends or family. They couldn't change the situation, they could only listen and I'm sure they were tired of hearing about this same issue over and over again from me. Even though I felt better temporarily when I would vent, the stress of the situation caused me to eat/snack while I would talk about my stressor. In addition, venting did not fix, and would not fix, the stressful situation I found myself in.

Addressing the Issue

When the one hour appointment took place between my boss and me, I had rehearsed my thoughts and was ready for our discussion. I had rehearsed my thoughts over and over and took the time in advance to list my issues (components). This kept me from losing my train of thought when meeting with him and not having me appear as an emotional woman—which unfortunately, is viewed negatively in the workplace.

I expressed to my boss how I felt, and I had examples of the inequities extended which of course included pay. Facts gave more credibility to my comments. My boss listened to all I had to say, questioned some of my facts, listened again to my perspective from being the only woman on the team, and then said he wanted to think about everything I said overnight. **I said all right, and that was my first step**

toward letting go. I listened to him as he had listened to me, instead of pushing for a resolution on the spot which I would have certainly done in the past.

From my alone time, I noticed that my pushing for immediate conclusions sometimes caused others to react negatively in meetings. What I found was that often they would come to the same conclusion as me but just not as fast. I needed to respect the way other people would think and give them enough time to process. It was a just a different style, not right, not wrong, just different. To make this a successful meeting, I was going to intentionally change my style. I realized that my boss' method of resolving an issue was to process the thoughts, where my personality was to come to an immediate conclusion.

I knew this as I had studied the four categories of personalities throughout my career but knowing something and actually practicing it, was different. This one step was a huge breakthrough in my behavior. **I had made a conscious effort to change me.**

In the morning my boss kept his promise and we met again. He told me he decided to make a substantial pay adjustment for me. He hadn't realized the disparity and was committed to fixing it. On the other issues, he expressed that he acknowledged what I had said, and that we all needed to consciously work together as a team and get along. This would make us all more successful.

I had finally resolved this issue by going to the one person who could resolve the problem. I am guessing that he talked confidentially to one or two of the other members of the team about their behavior, but I'm not positive about that. It didn't matter anymore, because at that point when I shared my anger, hurt, feelings of unfairness and examples, **with someone who could do something about it**, someone who was the right person in the proper chain of command, I was letting go. I didn't have to know what happened behind closed doors (it was not my business) and I didn't need to know every detail of the actions that led to the reaction.

I had to only acknowledge my feelings of being set free from this stress and having the others know that I would not be taken advantage of or treated differently, just because I was a woman. Whether the environment changed or not, I was releasing from my body all of the things that had been bottled up in me for over a year, hitting the conflict head on with the only person who could resolve the issue, and I then resolved to **let it go**. The stress was no longer bottled up in me and I was free to stay or leave voluntarily, but the unresolved stress would no longer eat away at me or cause me to eat. I could walk right past the community candy bowl now and not even be tempted to take a piece from it anymore!

I dropped three pounds that week and two pounds the next. I put an "X" over this stressor on my list. It was now eliminated from my life and I couldn't believe how much better I felt!

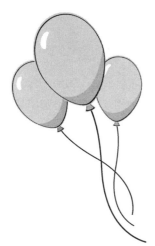

Chapter 10

Let's Try This Again

*T*he next stressor I chose was again work related. Since work issues are less personal and were truly just business, I found they were easier for me to resolve.

I was very hurt that Carol, the woman on my staff, had betrayed me numerous times behind my back. This had never happened to me before in all of the years that I had managed people, so it was a new experience for me. Trust is very important to me and is necessary to have in a business relationship, just as it is necessary to have in a personal relationship.

Trust is needed to keep a team or a relationship running at its best. A violation of trust in any situation, whether it's work or personal, is devastating.

I thought about the issue that had occurred with Carol, over and over, as to what I might have done to contribute to this behavior of betrayal. Then I thought about the personal make-up/background of the individual who was betraying me, and then how she contributed to our conflict.

After thinking it through, I realized that I had inherited Carol as a part of my staff when I joined the company. I did not interview or hand pick her to work for me. However, I went into the work situation openly with trust when I should have first observed and decided if I could trust this person before I blindly trusted with no proven history between us. That was my fault and that was how I contributed to this particular stress situation.

I had unintentionally set myself up for disappointment by not looking into the past behavior of this person. I just trusted from the beginning because she "looked" professional. This was my mistake which ended up causing a lot of conflict for me in my job as Carol tried to tear me down and all that I was working on, to save herself. After carefully investigating, I found that Carol was not qualified for the position that she was in and had fully realized this even before I did. She was prepared to do anything she could to preserve her salary since she was truly over paid for what she was actually contributing. As a result, she had moved into a survivor mode, trying to discredit me before the crash of self.

I became anxious due to the stress every day that we had to meet to discuss business items, since all of the trust between us had been destroyed. I had been hearing the comments she was making about me from numerous people in the company. People she trusted were coming to me behind her back repeating every negative word she said about me.

Everything is Repeated

In a work setting it is important to know that **everything you, or anyone else says, will be repeated.** How many times have you heard someone say "I'll tell you this but you have to promise to not tell anyone else." These are probably the same words someone else said to them. This is common in a business setting as everything said usually returns full circle, with an added tail.

All of Carol's back-stabbing and deceitful comments were being repeated back to me by her "trusted" sources. I was angry and hurt by my knowledge of her deceit, and as I became stressed from our meetings, I ate. The stress eating would start almost immediately after we met. As soon as she would leave my office I would make a quick dash for the always available candy dish. My anger and stress triggered something in me that only quickly accessible, high fat/high sugar foods would relieve.

Since I had previously shared my thoughts with my boss on the other issue that had been bothering me and there was a positive outcome, I once again went to him after I had thoroughly outlined my facts and plan.

I knew that Carol was not qualified for the job she held and the cost of her salary and benefits was substantial to the business. I recommended that her position be eliminated. The company would save the cost of the salary and benefits, and I would be eliminating from my life a person who was constantly providing me stress and who didn't deliver the results of the job that were expected.

My boss once again listened to all I had to say, accepted my proposal, and the position was eliminated as it truly was no longer needed in our business.

Once I moved myself away from the personal part of the equation and focused on the issue only as a business problem, the right answer came to me. Now another stressor had

91

been eliminated from my life and it was a tremendous relief to let that go.

Once I eliminated the position, I let go of all of the past hurts associated with her. I let it go and will not look back but I will change my behavior and not trust anyone until they first prove that they are trustworthy to me. This was an interesting, but tough, lesson for me to learn.

I lost five pounds from when I started to think about the problem until its conclusion. My total weight loss was now ten pounds. Since a loss of eight pounds usually makes a one size difference in clothes, I was starting to notice my clothes were getting a little bit too big. What a great feeling that is because **there is nothing that you can taste that will be as satisfying as seeing the new thin you in the mirror!**

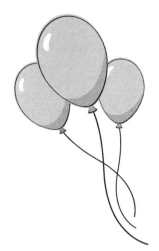

Chapter 11

Losing the Urge to Snack

*N*ow that I had lost ten pounds in weight, I found I had lifted ten pounds of stress from my body. I was not filling myself with high fat/high calorie food soothers as often as before, and I wasn't feeling as stressed as I had been before and therefore was not as hungry.

As I went grocery shopping, I tried to buy only fresh foods and avoided as much processed, packaged, and frozen foods as possible.

I decided to eat as much as I wanted, **without measuring**, of the following:

- ❏ Chicken (no skin)
- ❏ Lean Beef (Lean Hamburger and Steak)
- ❏ Meatballs (Homemade)
- ❏ Chile (no toppings)
- ❏ Pork Chops
- ❏ Fish (baked or broiled, not breaded)
- ❏ Shellfish
- ❏ Turkey or chicken lunchmeat

- ❑ Eggs or egg substitute, cooked in a variety of ways
- ❑ Canadian Bacon
- ❑ Peanut butter
- ❑ All fresh vegetables
- ❑ Salad (no cheese, croutons, or creamy dressings)
- ❑ All fresh fruits
- ❑ Sugar-free applesauce
- ❑ Lemons or limes squeezed on salad, fish, or chicken
- ❑ Soups (not creamy, only broth based)
- ❑ Salsa (No chips) on top of eggs, fish, or poultry
- ❑ BBQ Sauce on chicken, fish, or salad
- ❑ Mustard, Ketchup and Pickles are an acceptable accessory on food
- ❑ Whole wheat pasta with marinara (red) sauce or a little bit of olive oil with vegetables
- ❑ Fat-free yogurt (any flavor)
- ❑ Oatmeal
- ❑ Sugar free popsicles
- ❑ All fat free/sugar free instant puddings (any flavor), made with skim milk
- ❑ Whipped cream as a topping on fruit or pudding
- ❑ Caramel topping or chocolate syrup on fruit
- ❑ Diet soda, skim milk, plain iced tea and lots and lots of water.

To turn water into flavorful new beverages to consume, I would fill a pitcher with tap water to keep cool in the refrigerator and then alternate these items to add to each pitcher for a different flavor:

- ❑ lemon slices
- ❑ lime slices
- ❑ cucumber slices
- ❑ orange slices
- ❑ raspberries
- ❑ strawberries.

Experiment and use as much dry seasoning as you would like to change the flavor of chicken or fish. Explore new spices to create new flavors for your food and try to use a little bit of olive oil or vegetable spray when cooking.

By eating as much of these foods listed above whenever I wanted, I was full, satisfied, and amazingly not as hungry as I had been in the past. This was not a diet as I wasn't counting calories or measuring items. **This was a lifestyle change**.

I was also simultaneously removing the stressors out of my life which caused me to eat.

In addition, I noticed that I was not as bloated as I had been in the past. I think that was due to not eating processed foods loaded with preservatives and by eliminating cheese from my diet. Besides losing weight, having more energy, and not feeling bloated, my blood sugar levels were lowering on their own without any medication which was a healthy side benefit.

There were numerous meals I could make with these items listed above with lots of variation.

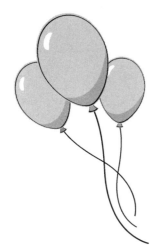

Chapter 12

Sample Menus While Letting Go

*L*isted on the following pages are sample menus incor-porating all of the "approved" foods you can eat for your first two weeks of Losing Weight by Letting Go.

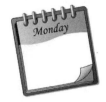

Monday

Breakfast   1 egg cooked over easy with vegetable spray, no butter, and one piece of Canadian bacon. Coffee or tea plain or with skim milk (no sugar or sugar substitute)

10 a.m.   1 banana

Lunch   Salad of any type with balsamic vinaigrette as the dressing. Any type of meat or seafood can be included, but no cheese or croutons. When dining out, always order the salad without cheese or croutons and your dressing served on the side. You will consume less dressing this way instead of having your salad served with the dressing already mixed in.

3 p.m.   One piece of fruit or individual serving of sugar free applesauce

Dinner   1 bowl of soup (not creamy) any kind

1 boneless/skinless chicken breast stir fried with fresh vegetables, topped with soy sauce

8 p.m.   Fat free, sugar free pudding made with skim milk, topped with a little spray of whipped cream

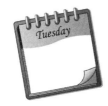

Tuesday

Breakfast Fat-free yogurt with fresh strawberries

10 a.m. 1 apple

Lunch Chili—all you want (<u>no</u> toppings, such as sour cream or cheese)

3 p.m. Fresh strawberries—as many as you want

Dinner Small steak broiled or grilled, roasted or grilled tomato slices seasoned with pepper, corn on the cob (roasted on the grill or boiled—no butter). If you take the corn out of the husk and place it directly on the grill to cook, it will roast slowly and be flavorful so you will not need to add butter.

8 p.m. 1 banana with fat free hot caramel sauce drizzled on top

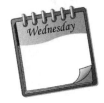

Wednesday

Breakfast   1 egg scrambled, coffee or tea plain or with skim milk

10 a.m.   1 banana

Lunch   Chicken Caesar salad (no croutons or cheese on top)

3 p.m.   Fresh fruit or sugar free applesauce

Dinner   Fresh fish grilled or baked in the oven with lemon, roasted cauliflower (wrap cauliflower in foil with a dab of olive oil, salt, pepper and garlic—roast at 450 degrees for 45 minutes)

8 p.m.   Sugar-free, fat-free pudding, any flavor

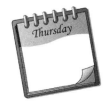

Thursday

Breakfast	Egg substitute mixed with stir-fried mushrooms to create a mini omelet.
10 a.m.	1 banana
Lunch	Taco salad (no cheese, no sour cream, and no tortilla bowl)
3 p.m.	Fresh fruit or sugar free applesauce
Dinner	Lettuce topped with grilled chicken breast (which had been marinated in teriyaki sauce), fresh avocado slices and chopped fresh tomatoes
8 p.m.	One cup sugar free cocoa blended with ice

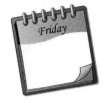

Friday

Breakfast   Fat free, sugar free pudding made with skim milk (any flavor) topped with whipped cream.

10 a.m.   One banana

Lunch   Grilled burger, preferably a turkey burger,* with lettuce, tomato, onion, mushrooms (no cheese, no bun)

Chicken broth soup with sliced mushrooms and small slices of green onions. (Add one teaspoon of soy sauce to the chicken broth to enhance the flavor.)

3 p.m.   Fresh fruit or sugar free applesauce

Dinner   Shrimp grilled or stir fried in a tablespoon of oil, with fresh sliced vegetables and seasoned with soy sauce

8 p.m.   A sliced apple dipped in fat free caramel sauce **or** bake a whole apple (cut off the top before baking and add one teaspoon of butter and sprinkle with cinnamon) for 30 minutes at 350 degrees. Drizzle with fat free caramel sauce after removing from the oven.

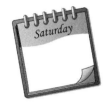

Saturday

Breakfast   Egg substitute omelet with fresh chopped tomatoes and green onions. Top with salsa if you like.

10 a.m.   Fresh strawberries—as many as you want

Lunch   Turkey lunchmeat rolled with lettuce, tomato and green onions plus a bowl of broth-based soup.

3 p.m.   Fresh fruit or sugar free applesauce

Dinner   Crab legs (cook crab legs in boiling water without salt), serve with fresh lemon slices (no butter), and sweet potato baked fries. (Cut a sweet potato into strips, spray with vegetable oil spray, sprinkle pepper lightly on top of the sliced sweet potato, bake 45 minutes at 450 degrees).

8 p.m.   Glass of wine or two, if you like

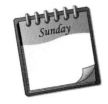

Sunday

Breakfast   1/2 Bagel with reduced fat cream cheese, spread thinly, any flavor. (The new 100 calorie bagels are tasty, filling, and are much lower in calories than other bagels).

10 a.m.   Fresh fruit—your choice

Lunch   Chopped salad (no cheese) tossed with balsamic vinaigrette—2 Tbs.

3 p.m.   Fresh fruit or sugar free applesauce

Dinner   Homemade meatballs**, red marinara sauce (jar sauce is fine) and whole wheat pasta

8 p.m.   Nothing tonight, you'll be too full

* **Turkey Burgers**—Before I changed my eating habits by letting go, the thought of eating a turkey burger was unappealing; in fact it just seemed like something I couldn't do—it just didn't seem right. They actually taste good and leave you feeling less full.

** **Homemade Meat Balls**—Mix one pound of lean ground been with one egg, a small sprinkle of pepper to taste, and add a sprinkle of oregano and one half cup of breadcrumbs. Roll into balls, and place on a foil lined baking sheet and bake for 20 minutes. Do not fry the meatballs ever again. Baking is an easier method to cook most food instead of frying and will save tons of calories by not using any oil to coat the pan.

After I was able to let go of the stress and started to reduce my high fat/high sugar food intake, other foods started to taste different to me. Things I once thought were delicious, like cheese, now were too heavy for my digestive system.

One day, my daughter Kay brought home a box of turkey burgers for us to try. Not for me, I thought. After she cooked the turkey burger on the grill, it looked like any other burger. I agreed to try one bite and was really surprised. It not only tasted like a "normal" hamburger, but when I was finished, it didn't leave that heavy feeling in my stomach. It was so much lighter due to having less calories and fat than beef burgers. All summer we changed from traditional hamburgers to turkey burgers and actually a few friends became hooked on them as well.

Any Day—Chocolate Treat

When you have a craving for chocolate, skip the candy or a brownie, and instead make this chocolate treat at home. Mix in a glass, two pumps of chocolate syrup with two squirts of whipped cream. Mix together and add chilled, unflavored club soda. This will taste like a chocolate soda treat and has barely any calories.

Or, if you are in the mood for a warm chocolate treat, cook one cup of fat free milk on top of the stove and add about eight chocolate chip morsels to it. Stir the milk as the chocolate melts and you have an easy to make, tasty hot chocolate treat that does not include any processed chocolate powder drink mix.

While on your stress relieving journey and diet/lifestyle change, feel free to drink wine or liquor as you normally would. Notice however, that you might feel the effects of alcohol much quicker than you had before because you are no longer eating significant portions of bread, heavy chips or other bagged snacks, or fried foods to absorb the liquor you are taking in. Plus, since you are starting to actually resolve issues, and let go of your stress, you are not using liquor to numb the pain from your hurts and anger.

Be careful of your liquor intake now so you do not drink more than you can handle. I personally found that my tolerance for liquor was now cut in half.

After your first two weeks of successfully completing your new method of eating only approved food items and no food accessories, you can start adding whole wheat bread, brown rice and plain potatoes back into your meals but on a limited basis.

Your Dining Habits

- **Never eat the bread from a bread basket in a restaurant**. Ask the server to bring you one piece of bread with your meal or have a small baked white or sweet potato, or rice, but no more than one of these items at the same meal. Start making choices to manage your meal and enjoy the main course.

- After your first two weeks, try to incorporate your bread type item in the morning with your breakfast instead of with dinner so that you are not eating so heavy at the end of the day.

In order to manage what you are eating when dining out at a restaurant, stick to these methods to change your eating behavior:

Fast Food Restaurants

- Only select a salad (dressing on the side and always fat free), chili (no sour cream added) or a baked potato (with no toppings) from the menu.

Regular Restaurants

- Always start with a small salad which you can ask to be served to you immediately, even before you place your order. Have the server bring your dressing on the side. You will use less dressing that way compared to what you would consume if the salad is already pre-mixed.

- Ask the server to not bring a bread basket to your table or ask that only one piece of bread be served to you. If you have to have bread, skip the butter or olive oil and parmesan cheese, (you won't miss it, it's a food accessory).

107

- Next, order your dinner from the appetizer section or split a regular-sized meal with someone else. Always ask to substitute a vegetable for the rice or pasta or potatoes that might come with the dish. In addition, when ordering a vegetable, ask the server to be sure it is steamed or stir fried, not pre-soaked in butter or oil.

- If you're selecting an appetizer, crab cakes are usually a healthy choice. Skip the accompanying sauce and top only with fresh-squeezed lemon juice. Avoid appetizers that are breaded and fried or include cheese.

Remember, you are the customer who is paying for the items that you select. **It is your choice and right to alter anything that is offered on a menu**. Do not feel obligated to choose something from a menu just the way it is listed. Take your time and shave off lots of unnecessary fat and calories and food accessories from your meal when dining out, other people do this all of the time.

A Buffet or Brunch

You may still eat at a buffet, and enjoy lots of food, but you will be making different selections from those you had selected in the past.

Buffets are usually designed to be set up in a certain order. They usually begin with all of the filling mayonnaise based salads, heavy breads like muffins, doughnuts and sweet rolls; all lined up at the start of the buffet with all of the protein/carved meats located at the end of the buffet.

The desserts are strategically placed in your view, so that as you are gliding past all of the different food choices you will be tempted to pick up a rich, filling dessert before you finish your meal.

This layout is done intentionally so that guests will fill up on the heavier, more fattening, less expensive items and not fill up on the higher cost protein items. That is why filling up your plate, finishing it, and getting a new plate is encouraged. The buffet is designed in this manner so that by the time the guest finishes two plates of inexpensive, high fat, food they will be too full to eat the expensive seafood and meats that are offered and the buffet has successfully been profitable.

On your next buffet visit, you will maneuver through the buffet backwards starting with the protein to fill your plate.

- Fill your plate with the carved beef and/or turkey and feel free to add some eggs if they are available.

- If you should stop at the omelet station, ask the chef to line the pan for the omelet with vegetable spray instead of lining the pan with the traditional ladle of oil. The chef will usually keep a can of vegetable spray under the counter for those people who request it. If you don't request the vegetable spray, you'll get a ladle full of oil which packs on pounds to your body and makes you feel full faster.

- When choosing ingredients to add to your omelet, request only vegetables to be added to the omelet, and remember you will not be adding any cheese! After a few weeks you will not even miss the taste of cheese; it's just a food accessory that you were used to adding to your food.

- Fill up on these items first, before you touch anything else on the buffet. You will find you will be too full to eat the filling fatty foods that are lined up at the beginning of the buffet.

Stop and Think

Better choices at a buffet include:

- Fresh eggs cooked in vegetable spray are a better choice than prepared eggs with cheese added.

- Scrambled eggs are a better choice than an omelet.

- Skip the bread, bagels, crackers, and sliced cheese or cheese cubes displayed and select the fresh fruit offered instead.

- Choose from the salads that do not have a creamy mayonnaise base.

- Fill up on meats that are not battered or fried.

- Chicken or Turkey are better choices than Beef and Pork.

- Remove the sauce from any fish or remove the skin from any chicken before eating.

- Choose fresh fruit or chocolate covered strawberries as your dessert.

By following these steps, you can enjoy a very large, full plate of food while dining at a buffet. When enjoying lunch or dinner at a buffet, my plate is loaded and the people I dine with are usually surprised that I can eat that much and keep my weight in check. If they look closer they will see how my food choices are better options than what they have selected.

Often I will see people trying to "diet" who are planning to eat just a salad. They accessorize their salad with shredded cheese and croutons and top it all off with a load of cream based dressing. At the end of the meal they are not satisfied with their meal and they have just consumed more fat and calories than a person who is not dieting and who has decided to make better food choices.

If you stick with this meal plan for two weeks, without cheating, you'll notice how different sugar or processed foods taste when you try them again. Things that you used to think tasted great will now taste different and unpleasant.

Processed foods will taste different than fresh and you'll find you will prefer to eat the fresh food *if* you continue to **eliminate stress from your life.**

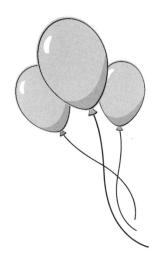

Chapter 13

The Stress of Family

I was now ten pounds lighter, and feeling much more energy, but the odd thing was that I was not as hungry as I had been before.

In the past, I was always nibbling. I was not really eating a lot of meals, but I was probably consuming more calories in my all day nibbling and snacking on high fat/high calorie foods than I did during my actual meals.

As I became less stressed, I was no longer reaching for the chocolate, nuts, chips, cheese sticks, etc. that were an immediate fix to calm me down. Hours would go by and I wouldn't even think of food or eating. Before I would eat a snack or a meal, I would notice that I was hungry, but I was no longer craving a particular food and I was starting to lose my taste for high fat/high sugar foods. All of a sudden one of my favorite outings, going out to dinner in a restaurant, had no longer become as much of an interest to me. I found I couldn't eat that much anymore and be comfortable. It now had become a natural habit to control myself to not touch the bread basket when I was dining out. Plus, I was starting to get interested in buying clothes again, now that I had lost some weight.

I was now ready to tackle stressor #3. It was time to eliminate the stress my daughter was causing me and the damage I felt she was causing herself.

Addressing Conflict

Sometimes it's so much easier to ignore a conflict situation and keep busy with work, chores and outside activities, rather than hit the conflict head on, but that does not resolve anything. Even though my child was 20 years old, and was becoming wonderfully independent, I felt it was my job as a parent to counsel her on the affects of excessive alcohol and the damage it could cause. At least the issue wasn't drugs; so many parents I knew were faced with horrible situations and stress when their kids became involved in drugs.

Since my daughter was tired of hearing me "preach", or nag as she would call it, she was avoiding any alone time with me. In the past we would spend lots of time together. One of our favorite activities was to take a long, fast, power walk and talk. It was our activity, and it used to be a good way for us to get exercise and catch up on what was going on in each other's life. Now, things had changed and in her eyes I was a mother who must have been born at age 40 and didn't realize that everyone in college drank.

One day the stress peaked to an erupting level and I couldn't hold in my frustration any longer. I felt like I was going to explode over Elle's behavior and I knew I had to address the drinking issue I was avoiding.

I took the opportunity to suggest that we get some fresh air. We went for a long walk one day and when we were about a half hour from our home, where she couldn't escape from me or my comments, I started expressing my thoughts/concerns/wisdom about the effects of alcohol and reiterated stories of "good judgment" to her. I intentionally waited to talk to her about our "conflict" until we were far from home because I was afraid that if I started this discussion as soon as we left the house, she would turn around and leave me rather than discuss it.

I had consciously adjusted my style in preparation for this talk. At first she resisted, then listened, and finally acknowledged her weaknesses. I had to give her some hard facts and examples of people we knew who let alcohol excess ruin their life. I didn't want her to be one of them.

At that point, I told her all that I had to say and that I was going to **"let go"** and hope that the 20 years of advice and counseling that I had given to her would stick. I would always be there for her, but it was time to trust her and her judgment. I had warned her of every possible reaction that any negative action could produce. I was concerned for her health and for her future.

We both survived her trip and she grew up from the independence and exposure of being on her own in Europe for ten days.

My growth was in seeing it had become time to **"Let Go"**.

My daughter was no longer a child and I had completed my job as a parent and I knew I had done my job well.

The stress I was carrying by being an over-protective parent had to stop. As hard as it was going to be, I needed to switch my role as a mother from "controller" to an advisor, when asked. Letting go of control is very hard but it is needed to maintain a solid relationship.

If control isn't stopped, a person or a relationship cannot grow naturally. When there is too much control, the conflict could cause a permanent split in the relationship. This should be avoided for the sake of saving a relationship that is important.

During my alone time, when I was breaking down this problem into components, I realized that I was being an over protective parent because I had been raising these children on my own for so long. As a single parent I was providing the advice, counsel, and control of both a mother and a father, and that is exhausting for one person.

When I accepted the fact that my child, now 20, could make it through life on her own without me, I lost another five pounds.

I had now lost 15 pounds and my clothes were all too big. The sense of calm I was moving towards was tremendous. I had crossed three items off my stressor list and was ready to tackle another.

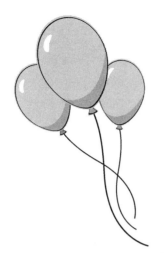

Chapter 14

The Stress of an Ex

I reviewed my list of stressors to see which one I had some control over to change/remedy and which one caused me the most stress.

I again took some quiet time to determine how I could still be battling with my ex-husband (we'll call him X) over child support/college expenses and his lack of participation in the parenting of our three daughters.

X and I had been divorced for 14 years now and my complaints were the same today as they were over the last 14 years; nothing had changed. We had been in court at the time of our divorce, we were in court six years later for child support adjustments, and we were back in court again six years after that.

When we actually got divorced we kept the process somewhat amicable. However, as the years went by and things became more costly, I became extremely resentful that he didn't participate in raising the kids, or taking them for weekends or holidays to give me any free time. Also, as his salary increased through the years he did everything he could to avoid increasing his child support payment. He felt, that any time he wrote a check to me for child support, that it was "fun money" for me. He had no idea or did he care, of how expensive it was to raise children.

The Final Straw

The final issue that caused me to explode from stress was the conversation that X and I had when one of our children needed braces. I wrote him a note telling him the minute monthly amount that we would need to split (per our divorce agreement). Since we were no longer speaking, sending notes kept us from screaming at each other.

His return note to me was "I'm not going to pay anything towards the braces. If you want; sue me." It was the final straw, all that I could take after raising the children, paying for their school and expenses, paying for their medical and dental coverage, and working full time—and so a lawyer was hired and the fight began. This time it had become a full blown battle. This stress had to stop as well as our constant bickering. We knew each others hot buttons and we continued to push them even after 14 years!

I finally realized that I was wasting all of my time, energy, and finances (by paying lawyers) to try and change someone who would never change. Plus, I finally realized that it was not my business or right to try and change my ex-husband.

I knew that fundamentally I was right, that he should share in the responsibilities of our daughters with me, but in my efforts to prove that I was right, the stress toll on me was tremendous. If he hadn't helped me with raising the kids over the last 12 years, **I should have let it go** and moved on instead of continuing the fight for the next two years.

As I spent more time reflecting on our issues, I focused on my weight fluctuations. I had always been thin as a child, teenager, college student, and then young adult. It wasn't until I was married about eight years that I started to put on some extra weight.

I blamed having children at that time and what it does to your body, but as I continued to reflect back, **the weight I gained was due to the stress in my marriage, not due to having children.**

The marriage had many problems probably starting in about year seven, which became increasingly worse for the next six years until I finally couldn't take it any more and asked for a divorce. The stress level I felt for those six years was incredible and I guess I **filled my loneliness with food as a comfort**. I wanted and had thought about getting a divorce every day for three years before I actually said the words.

Holding that thought in for three years and not sharing it with anyone, even friends or family, was a huge stressor to me. Even though the marriage was dead in the house, whenever we would be around friends or family we would put on such a believable act of getting along. It was always "Honey this, or honey that"... I'm not sure why we did that but we did, both of us. Then as soon as we were alone it was either silence or fighting—nothing in-between.

As much as I wanted to be out of the marriage and knew I wasn't happy, I was afraid to be on my own with three small children. Even though I had a well paying job and benefits, I didn't think I could handle it all alone without a spouse.

If I was afraid to make a move, I could only imagine how many women or men who did not have a good job or benefits felt trapped in a bad marriage and thought that they had no way out—and how stressed they must be.

When I finally made up my mind to take action and insisted on splitting up, the divorce process was quick; it was over in six months.

My husband moved out and my excess weight seemed to melt off. I went from a size 12 to a size 8 without dieting.

I thought at that time that it was from the stress of the divorce and the anticipation of raising my children alone, but as I look back, the weight loss was from **Letting Go**— letting go of a bad situation that would never work—letting go of a fantasy of a perfect marriage and household like you would see on TV, letting go of pretending to family, friends and neighbors, that it was a successful marriage when behind closed doors, it was not.

Although it was frightening not knowing what was ahead, this first step was liberating.

Being in my marriage I felt like I was trying to swim and someone was holding my legs; I couldn't move and was almost drowning.

Six years went by and my ex-husband and I were bickering again.

As I tried to get him to see my point of view and the expense and responsibility of raising three children, we argued, argued and argued. And I gained my weight back again. It came back slowly and I thought it was due to travel, a sedentary job, age or anything else I could blame it on except for stress.

Finally, after 14 years, I came to the realization that **you can't change someone else. People can only change if they personally want to**.

I finally realized I couldn't change him to meet <u>my</u> expectations of what a father should do or be like. I needed to let go, cease communication and forget about financial help for college.

I made up my mind that I would do this on my own which would be less stressful than ever trying to get him to understand and participate the way that I expected him to. It would be easier for me to take on the role of two parents than to try and ever get him to be the father that I wanted for my daughters.

I needed to accept him for who he was, accept his parenting for what it was, and let go and quit trying to change him into someone he would never be.

I needed to let go and be thankful that our union produced three great kids. I needed to put all of my energy into positive methods for me to continue raising and providing for my children on my own. Trying to control his behavior was a waste of time and energy for me and I had been doing it for too long.

When I made my decision to **Let Go**, an inner peace came over me that is so hard to describe. The anger, the anxiousness, the nervousness I had been feeling was now evaporating which was allowing the toxins from my body to exit.

I contacted my lawyer and said that we were finished; that we were not going to move forward with another motion, order, ruling, etc. She disagreed with me and said we were right and that we needed to continue to pursue the action. She said we could win this battle and years of back pay and support. If not the first time around, we would be sure to win on appeal.

I told her I knew we were right, but that I was Letting Go.

The anger/stress and waste of time and energy was no longer important to me. I had lost enough time, energy and money on this already. I should have Let Go years ago. I finally realized you can't change someone else no matter if you yell, cry, threaten, go to court, etc.

Even when you're right—that doesn't mean someone else will agree to do the right thing.

Change can only come from within and I was changing because I wanted to.

I would never be able to change him to see my point of view, to pay half of the college expenses, to attend parent/teacher conferences or weekend sporting events, to stay in on the weekends to supervise teenagers in the basement, to help with homework or teach them to drive. Plus, I was no longer going to try.

I wasn't sure how I would pay for all of the upcoming college expenses, but I had faith that **through honesty and integrity, I would find a way**. I would no longer worry about it; I was Letting Go of the hurts in my marriage, the hurts of my divorce and the ongoing hurts and insults in our battles post divorce.

When I made this decision to really **Let Go**, I lost ten more pounds and scratched one more stressor off my list. The weight kept dropping off effortlessly. I noticed I wasn't very hungry throughout the day and I became full with much smaller portions. I didn't have cravings. I sometimes forgot to eat and when I did eat, the natural foods like fruit, salad, fish and meats all tasted better to me.

Since I had eliminated so much stress from my life, I was much calmer, happier, relaxed and now had lost 25 pounds.

I was purchasing new items slowly as I was afraid each morning that I would wake up and the weight would return overnight.

It has been nearly two years now that I have let go and lost weight. My weight fluctuates about five pounds at the most.

I eat what I want, when I want, but fresh foods taste the best. I don't overeat and I don't buy or eat any food accessories anymore and I don't miss them.

I splurge a little on the weekend when dining out, but eliminating the food accessories from my plate has now become as natural as cutting up food before eating it. The better food choice list found in the appendix helps me to maintain my weight loss. These better food choices can cut lots of calories from your diet.

I realize the rest of my life will not be stress free, but when a huge stressor comes into my life, I am going to follow my own outlined steps of:

- Spending some time alone
- Break the new stressor down into components/steps to identify the whole picture of why this situation is so stressful to me
- Reflect on how I contribute to the stress and how others contribute to it
- Figure out how I can resolve the stressor and Let It Go from my life before it overtakes me.
- Follow my own action steps to **let it go**.

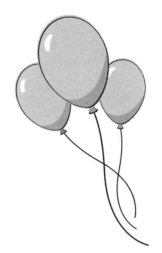

Chapter 15

Crossing Paths—
Stories from Others

*W*hen I was in the final stages of writing this book, and would meet someone new, the first thing this person would ask me is what I did for a living. I would reply that I was taking a year off from my human resources and consulting work to write a book.

When I would mention the title of the book I was writing, the response was enthusiastic and always the same.

People wanted to hear more about my book and immediately became intrigued and asked for more details.

When I would tell these individuals how **I lost weight by letting go of my stress,** they would then open up and start to share what had been bothering them, how stress or stressful issues caused them to eat non-healthy foods, and how badly they wanted to lose weight. They wanted to lose weight for a variety of reasons; not only for their appearance, but also for their health.

Interestingly, there was not one person that I discussed the topic of the book with who did not share at least one thing in their life that caused them to over eat and gain weight.

People of all sizes and shapes, no matter if they wanted to lose 10 pounds or 100 pounds, all agreed that much of their improper eating was due to the emotional stress in their life. In addition, even when the book was in its creative conceptual format, these people wanted to buy it!

From the sales clerks at the grocery store, to the people that helped me with copying and shipping at Fed Ex/Kinko's, to servers I would talk to in restaurants, or people I would sit next to on an airplane, everyone both male and female, seemed interested in this approach to eliminate stress.

Even the very thin and fit people, especially men, openly discussed the enormous amounts of stress in their life. They too were anxious to follow the steps in my book to learn how to conquer and eliminate the stress in their life, even though they didn't have any weight to lose!

I was starting to accumulate business cards as some of those people asked me to contact them as soon as the book was ready for purchase. I thanked all of them as their positive enthusiasm kept me committed to writing and finishing this book. If this book can help someone else, I've truly found my purpose.

Listed below are some of the stories that I heard during my writing journey:

Maryann

Maryann was a single woman in her 30's; very smart and highly educated. She held a professional position and did very well at work. She had never been married but she did hope to get married and have children at some point in her life. This was something that was important to her.

At this time, Maryann was involved in a serious relationship with a man who was divorced and about 10 years older then she was.

They had been together for about three years and she shared how the relationship had constant bouts of verbal abuse. Her partner kept her involved in his life and occupied almost all of her free time on his terms.

She would have to drive to his house, stay at his house, and help him with his business on the weekends. In return, she had a steady relationship that she hoped would soon end up in marriage. He would not commit to a future with her but kept her near by, telling her how great everything was just as is.

Maryann was the giver and her boyfriend was the taker in this relationship.

After one or two drinks he would become verbally abusive to her. His insulting comments and the affect they had on her caused her to eat constantly, reinforcing her boyfriend's control over her and making her feel worthless.

Every time he insulted her or called her a name, she ate. She felt so bad about her appearance that she stayed with him thinking no one else would want her. When he was completely sober, he was not a great partner, but he was not abusive. The feeling of being loved in the day and abused in

127

the evening kept this smart woman from leaving him to pursue her goal of having a loving partner and a family.

We both knew the steps she needed to take. She was pretty and smart and didn't deserve to be called names. She needed to leave him as he would never change.

Jackie

Jackie, a divorced mom in her 40's, said that she was arguing with her ex-husband about him watching their children on the weekend so that she could work.

Jackie's job wasn't a typical Monday through Friday position. She was an in demand make-up artist who was called upon at all hours of the day or night when there was a photo shoot or a film in production.

Her "X" did not want to be bothered with their children on "his" weekends.

Every time Jackie was required to work on a Saturday or Sunday she would feel the apprehension building knowing that she would have to ask her ex for help with the kids. She couldn't afford to hire someone to help, she needed to work, and she couldn't get her ex-husband to understand that parenting was a joint responsibility—even on the weekends. She was eating constantly because of the stress and their constant arguing.

Jackie could either continue to use up her energy arguing with her ex-husband for the next few years or she could find a different solution to her problem that wouldn't cause her as much stress. She needed to realize that he was not going to change so she needed to spend some quiet time alone to search for her solution.

Monica

Monica, a hard worker who was happily married, shared that she was self employed and was working full-time running her business. Her husband had been employed steadily, but he had just lost his job.

Monica and her husband had their health insurance benefits through his company and now they weren't sure if they would be able to find any other health coverage since they both had minor medical problems—and she ate from the stress.

The extra weight that Monica was gaining was only making her current health problems worse. They had plenty of savings so money was not a factor. **She was focusing on, and stressing over, something that hadn't even taken place yet!**

Since they had the opportunity to buy COBRA, the extended medical coverage from his employer for the next 18 months, there was no need to stress about this issue today.

Monica needed to break their problem down into multiple steps (components) and focus on the long term solution, not just worry about the immediate problem.

Jeff

Jeff, a really, really, nice guy in his early 50's, was someone who always tried to please everyone in his life.

A good hearted guy, Jeff loved spending time with his wife and children and he enjoyed spending time with his parents as well. He told me that his parents, who were now in their 80's, had fallen ill.

Jeff told me he was in a fairly new position at work and under tremendous stress to perform. In addition to his long work day and two hour commute, his schedule changed constantly. He tried to spend quality time with his own family. He also wanted to take the time to see his parents and help with their care even though they lived almost an hour away from him. He was so tired and stressed that he didn't feel like he had enough energy to care for his wife, children, or parents.

In addition, Jeff was smoking cigarettes again. He ate very unhealthy as he was always on the run, putting himself last.

We talked about how he needed to take control of the job and not let it control him, and how he would need to get some help from other family members. He had to start by taking care of himself or he would not be healthy enough to care for everyone else in his life.

Katherine

Katherine was a young woman that I met on an airplane. She was newly engaged and in her mid 20's. She expressed that she was in a job that was not fulfilling plus it didn't pay well. She felt that she couldn't quit this job because some pay was better than no pay, and she had so many wedding expenses looming ahead of her.

This soon to be bride ate from the stress and felt terrible about the weight she was gaining as she wanted to look her best for the wedding.

We talked about how she needed to let go of the thought that this would be the only job she would ever have. She was young and healthy and had her whole future in front of her. She needed to think of what she would do if her job was eliminated tomorrow. When she decided what those steps were, those were the steps she needed to take to obtain a new job.

Donna

Donna, a woman in her late 50's, shared that her only son had died suddenly from an unexpected illness and the grief she was experiencing was overwhelming.

The weight gain was the result of this stress and knowing that her life would never be the same or as happy as it was in the past. The pain from her grief was so strong that you could feel it just being near her.

My heart went out to Donna as she had experienced every parent's worst nightmare. The only steps I could offer her were to suggest that she seek out a grief support group to share her feelings with. She needed to let go of trying to change the past which she couldn't do, and just focus on the wonderful memories and move forward with the loved ones who needed her so much now.

It would not be easy and her life would never be the same, but maybe through the support group she could find some peace and relief of stress.

Lynn

Lynn was a woman I met at a neighborhood party. She was healthy and in her late 40's, and was married to a very successful man named Rob. Lynn commented that she felt like she was a single parent with an income. Rob's constant travel and work left all of the home related duties and child rearing to her alone. Hoping she was always making the right decisions, she ate from the stress and never had time for herself.

Although Lynn did not have much weight to lose, the little bit of extra weight that she carried in her mid-section kept her feeling negative about herself. No one else noticed this and most people thought she looked fabulous for her age. Her stress level caused her to have a poor body image that wasn't even true.

After thinking her issues through, Lynn decided that she needed to schedule some time with her husband on a weekly basis to discuss family issues. This would help her by giving her a forum to share the concerns she had associated with raising a family. She needed her partner to listen and discuss their family issues and share in the decision making responsibilities.

Stephanie

Stephanie, a college student, was under pressure to go to school and work two jobs to help contribute to her school expenses. The worry and stress as well as her hectic schedule caused her to eat unhealthy and gain weight.

Stephanie needed to make some time for herself and pack a healthy lunch. She needed to stop purchasing high fat accessories like chips and candy when she was on the go. She was misguided into thinking that she wasn't eating much food, when in fact the little bit that she did eat was unhealthy and loaded with fat and calories.

This stressed student would have more energy if she would eat properly and consume more fruit and vegetables. Her diet needed to include something substantial mid-day like a turkey sandwich (no mayo!) to help her stay energized during for school and work.

Barbara

Barbara relayed that she was overeating and carrying stress weight because her husband was not working. The whole family's financial burden fell on her shoulders. She ate unhealthy food constantly from the stress and responsibility that she felt.

However, in order to avoid weight gain, she was purging once a day after a large meal. This destructive cycle was starting to take a serious toll on her body, her looks, and her health. Purging can damage your teeth and organs so this method of self-destruction had to be addressed.

The first steps Barbara needed to identify in her alone time was why her husband wasn't working, why he wasn't looking for a job, and why she allowed this situation to continue in her household. Once she focused on what the real problem was, she would find a solution.

Tony and Denise

Tony and Denise were a very devoted couple, with one child. I met them through the parents association at school. They were experiencing tremendous stress as their college student had become heavily involved in drugs.

As a couple, they did not make much money but they were very happy together. They had been married for a long time and really enjoyed each other. They borrowed extensively to send their only son away to college, out of state. The devastating result was that their son wasted the money and got involved with the wrong crowd and drugs.

They had to take a tough stand and pull him out of school. The arguments at home were taking a toll on their marriage. Their retirement money was now gone, they had additional debt building up and they both gained weight from the stress.

Tina

Tina, a woman who was married for 5 years and in her early 30's, found out she could not have children. This devastating news made her sad, then angry, and caused her to reach out to food for comfort. Her entire life she had planned on having a family and this news was devastating to her.

Infidelity

Both men and women of varying ages commented on how they found out that their spouse was cheating on them.

The stress from the break in the circle of trust was devastating and the heart break and stress caused many to eat. Each one who said their initial suspicions were guided by their gut—were the ones who ate to quiet this inner conscience.

Secrets

Anne said she became pregnant as a teenager. The pregnancy was unplanned and neither she nor the father was prepared for this responsibility. They agreed that she should have an abortion. They never discussed the issue with their parents or any other adults. They tried to solve the issue quickly, in the way they thought best.

Thirty years had gone by and Anne was now married to someone else and had a family. Her secret guilt from this experience has caused her to maintain extra weight because she never allowed herself to be forgiven for the choice she made so long ago.

Abuse

Tony, an alcoholic, shared how much anger and guilt he was carrying through the years because he watched his father be abusive to his mother. He was young and didn't know what to do at the time. His mother died at an early age and he felt she just gave up on life. He carried this weight as a memory along with his other addictions.

Money and Power

Sam was successful, extremely wealthy, yet consumed by the lawsuit he was in with of all people, his son. The father and son were battling over millions of dollars and it was all Sam could talk about to anyone who would listen. He ate and drank constantly and his belly was swollen from too much stress and too much liquor. He said he would fight this battle no matter what it cost him. I told him to let it go before the battle killed him. What good would his millions be then?

Family

Jen is a young woman in her late twenties that I have known since she was a ten years old. She has a very large family that is over protective of her, but they truly want the best for her.

The family continuously interferes in her love life finding something wrong with every man she dates. Her latest boyfriend ended up getting into a huge argument with her family which caused them to break up. The family was thrilled but it left Jen feeling very lonely and sad; so she cried and ate.

Jen wanted to get back together with her boyfriend but she knew how her family felt about him. Plus, they had given her an ultimatum in anger that she needed to pick either him or them. She continued to eat from the stress.

After a few months, Jen started to see her old boyfriend again and just failed to mention it to her family. Sneaking around and keeping this secret from the family she loved so much caused her so much stress and anxiety that she kept gaining weight. Since she was in love, she was too blind to see the flaws in her partner that her family could see clearly.

However, she was an adult and they needed to realize that they couldn't protect her forever.

Sometimes you have to let go and let your kids make mistakes in order for them to learn and grow.

Accepting the Truth

Pat was a woman I met who openly shared that her weight gain and stress was all due to the fact that her husband of seven years broke her heart and told her he was gay.

The stress came because she truly loved him and thought they had a good marriage. It was her second marriage and she was thrilled that she found love a second time around. He had helped heal her heart from her first divorce and she was very grateful to him for that. They spent lots of time together and shared many common interests.

When he came out, he admitted that he did love her but he was tired of pretending to be someone he was not. He had a male lover on the side and no longer wanted to keep up the charade.

Pat was devastated and took lots of steps to heal, but the stress of the situation was too much for her and she remained extremely over weight. She needed to identify what was truly bothering her, let it go, and not blame herself in any way for his sexual preference. She needed to realize that his sexual preference had been determined long ago and had nothing to do with her.

Let It Go

Secrets, guilt, grief, heartbreak, anger, verbal and physical abuse, lack of confidence; all of these are items that cause us to eat. It is time to get relief and start conquering these items by letting go of the past and focusing on the future.

A change in attitude, a change in job, a change in lifestyle, or a change in the people you surround yourself with can change your life, your outlook, and your weight.

In each situation where someone shared, I wanted to reach out and help.

For every single person who crossed my path by chance and felt comfortable enough to open up and tell me about their stress and the weight gain associated with it, I applaud your honesty. **That is the first step in letting go.**

The next step for each person to take is to identify their stressors.

Follow that by then breaking each of these stressful situations into small, manageable steps to attack and conquer.

Work on setting yourself free from the weight of stress.

I think that it helped all of these people that I took the time to listen. I listened to what they had to say and what was hurting them.

Hopefully, they will **lose weight by letting go.**

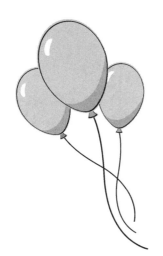

Chapter 16

You Can't Change Someone Else

*I*n conclusion, in your own life, there will be people you want to change. It could be a parent, sister, brother, spouse, boyfriend, girlfriend, an ex, work associate, boss, neighbor, etc.

You cannot change any of them so stop trying or wishing they would change; they won't.

Change yourself and accept that other person for whom he or she is, then decide if it's beneficial or hurtful to have that person in your life.

If it's beneficial, accept that person for who they are, love them just the way they are and do not try to change them. Appreciate them for who they are and what they add to your life.

If the relationship is hurtful or abusive, verbally or physically, if it makes you doubt yourself or feel bad about yourself, or your morals, values, and ethics are too different, you need to let go of the relationship to help yourself heal.

If it is a family member that is causing you to lose your self-confidence or causing stress in your life, you might need to put space between you and that person for a while so that you can feel better about yourself. Just because someone is a relative doesn't mean that the relationship is good for you.

When you finally Let Go, you will start to lose the excess pounds you are carrying. This happens first by first letting go of the weight of emotional pain which in turn releases the body weight. If you control your stress and pay attention to what you eat, you will be able to maintain a healthy weight.

Get healthy, stay happy, and **enjoy your life**. Wake up every day and be thankful for what you have, and pray for what you want. This really works. Put God, yourself, your spouse or significant other, family and friends first, your job second, and your chores third.

This will give you a life in order with the right rewards coming to you. Your house might be messy and your laundry might be backed up, but your relationships will be better and that makes for a much more rewarding life. Jobs and careers are rewarding and a paycheck makes life easier, but if the primary focus is work, the relationship area suffers.

Always be kind to other people; it is the right thing to do.

In addition, you never know what trauma or pain someone you meet might have in their life. So much happens behind closed doors that we surely shouldn't judge anyone else. If everyone would be a little bit nicer, a little bit more generous, and show a little more kindness, we could make life a little easier for everyone else.

Listed on the next page are a few things to start with on your journey of being a good person:

- Hold the door open for the person behind you even when you don't know them

- Never park in a handicap spot unless you're legitimately disabled

- Say "I love you" not "Love You" often

- Be sure to kiss your family good-bye in the morning

- Donate as much as you feel comfortable in giving to charity, and then give a little more

- Donate in front of your children so the lesson stays with them.

- Compliment other people all of the time. Find the best feature someone has and notice it. Compliment people of all sizes, shapes, and all ages

- Do not use your car horn unless it's a life threatening situation

- Never get up close behind another car because you're late or angry

- Make time to play with your dog or cat

- Say hi to strangers you pass on the street

- Acknowledge service workers by name when they wear a name tag

- Treat animals kindly

- Smile

- Count to ten before you yell at your kids

- Take out the garbage when its not your turn

- Buy coffee or lunch for someone unexpectedly

- Give an elderly person a ride if you see they are waiting for a bus

- Donate used clothes to a battered women's shelter or homeless shelter

- Donate used towels and bedding to an animal shelter

- Mentor a teenager

- Drive a friend to the airport

- Cook a meal for someone

- Volunteer one day per month for a charity or join a non-profit board

- Make your kids volunteer at least one day per month

- Take time for your friends and make sure you are selecting friends that are as good to you as you are to them

- Stop being angry at an ex-husband or ex-wife; you loved that person at one time so remember all of the good memories and let go of the bad ones

- Be nice to kids, they are the future

- Be respectful

- Don't make a joke at someone else's expense

- Don't text while driving or walking

- Tip generously when you have had good service

- Don't litter

- Smile

- Say Thank You often

- Go green — save energy when you can

- Recycle

- Keep a cloth bag in your car to carry groceries

- Do not use foam cups or plates
- Write thank you notes
- Give someone a $5 gift card when they do something nice or special for you; it's the thought not the value, that counts
- Let out of town friends stay at your home instead of a hotel
- Mentor someone
- Tell the truth
- Drop off some groceries at a food bank
- When a car puts on a blinker to enter your lane, let them in
- Pray for peace
- Stay in school
- Help someone out of work get a job
- Be nice to foreigners; you might be in their country some day and hope that someone will be nice to you
- Don't laugh at inappropriate jokes that you don't find funny just to fit in with the crowd
- If your meal tastes bad, don't take it out on the server
- If you know someone who is alone, invite that person to your holiday dinners
- Show respect and admiration for our military men and women; invite them to your holiday dinner if you live near a base
- Always stop and buy a drink when a child has a lemonade stand open; encourage the entrepreneur!

- Listen when your child or teenager has something to tell you

- Try not to multi-task; you will miss the moment.

My body is back to where it supposed to be given my age. No surgery, no pills, gimmicks or tricks; just eating the natural food that God provides for me. The formula is simple, yet you can't follow it unless you're ready to Let Go.

Let go of the past and look forward to the future. And if you've ever gone through a divorce or a significant break up, no matter how long ago it was, I recommend you find a Divorce Recovery Program at your community church and attend at least one eight-week session, if not more.

Several months ago, I saw my sister who had been out of the country for a year. The greatest compliment she could ever give me was when she pulled me aside and asked me if I secretly had liposuction. "Absolutely Not!" I told her, with a huge smile on my face. All I did was let go.

Two weeks ago, I stopped in to see an old friend who is a jeweler. We see each other about once every three months. He asked me if I had some work done on my face. "What do you mean?" I asked. He said, "I mean plastic surgery, you look great!" I told him, "No I didn't, I just let go." He looked at me strangely, not sure what I meant but I knew the stress that I used to carry around was now gone.

Just remember, when you feel the stress of a situation start to control you or your emotions, make a decision to **LET IT GO** before it takes hold of you.

PEACE

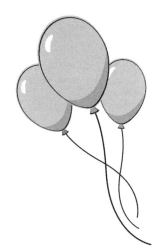

Appendix I

Places Where You Should Not Eat

- ❑ On an airplane
- ❑ In a movie theatre
- ❑ In a classroom
- ❑ In your office
- ❑ In your bed
- ❑ In the car
- ❑ On a walk
- ❑ At a concert
- ❑ In front of the TV
- ❑ On a bus or train
- ❑ In front of the computer
- ❑ At your desk

We have been conditioned to eat at many of the places listed above. It is not because we need to eat in any of those places but we are conditioned to do so throughout our life.

Most movies are less than two hours in length and most theatre productions are no more than three hours. Movies and theatre productions offer food and drink to increase their business revenue while at the same time adding excess weight to the patrons. It is unlikely that you need to eat or drink for the two or three hours spent in the movie theatre or while watching a play. This is a habit you will now break and it will also cause you to save money.

Eating on an airplane is also a habit, not a necessity, unless you are diabetic or have low blood sugar. If a flight is four hours or less, you should eat something healthy before you get on the plane and eat something healthy when you get off. The last minute food choices offered at the airport and on-board are not healthy alternatives. You would be better off to prepare ahead of time for the trip and have a meal before you get to the airport. Find another activity such as reading, sleeping, working, or identifying your stressors, to keep you occupied when on a plane instead of eating.

You need to realize that eating while driving is not safe. There is a possibility of a choking hazard if you should have to stop suddenly or if someone hits your car unexpectedly; plus, it is a bad habit to teach your children to eat in the car.

Never bring food into your bedroom. This should be your peaceful sanctuary for rest and intimacy.

Try not to eat while in your office, at your computer, or while watching TV. All of these activities take time and need your attention. If you are eating while working, you are not savoring the meal you are eating and might overeat because you are not paying attention to the food but rather your work you are doing or the television show you are watching.

Places you should eat a meal or snack would be at the kitchen or dining room table, or outside at a table, or on a blanket when having a picnic. Another option is to sit down in a restaurant for a snack or a meal. To keep our eating habits appropriate, we should take the time to enjoy our meal properly and not make it a part-time activity while doing something else. Dining is a great experience and we need to make the time to do it properly.

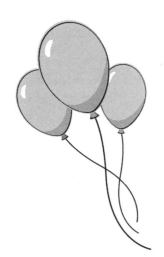

Appendix II

New Lifestyle/Better Food Choices

Some people have never been taught just what a good food choice is versus a bad food choice. It can be very easy to eliminate lots of pounds from your body by selecting healthier food choices while and after you are LETTING GO.

Choice	Better Choice
Cappuccino	Coffee with skim milk
Coffee with cream or half and half	Coffee with skim milk
Use skim milk at home and you will get used to the taste. When eating out in a restaurant, do not use the non-dairy creamers on the table but request skim milk or 2% from the server for your coffee. You have the right to ask for this.	
Milk	Skim milk
Pop/Soda	Diet Pop/Diet Soda
You will get used to the taste of diet soda after a few days. You will be cutting lots of calories from your diet just by making this better choice.	

Choice	Better Choice
Diet Pop/Diet Soda	Water
Increase your water intake and break the habit of always ordering coffee or pop when out in a restaurant. Water cleanses the system and our body needs it to function properly. In addition, you will save money.	
Sweetened Tea	Unsweetened Tea
Stop adding sugar, you will lose your taste for it	
Large glass of juice	Small glass of juice
Small glass of juice	Glass of Club Soda with a splash of juice
Beer	Light Beer
Omelet	Scrambled Eggs
(mix with water instead of milk in a pan coated with vegetable spray)	
Quiche	Eggs, any style
Bacon or Sausage	Canadian Bacon
Whole Bagel	One half of a Bagel
Doughnut	One half of a Bagel
Sugar Coated Cereal	Non-Sugar Coated Cereal
Croissant	1/2 English Muffin
Candy	Popcorn, no butter
Beef or Pork Ribs	Steak or Pork Chop
Steak or Pork Chop	Chicken or Turkey
Fried Chicken	Baked Chicken
Chicken or Turkey	Fish or Shellfish
Tuna packed in oil	Tuna packed in water
Fried Foods	Broiled or Baked Foods
Mayonnaise Based Salads	Garden Salad with Fat Free Dressing
Creamy Dressing	Vinaigrette Dressing
Dressing on the Salad	Dressing on the Side

Choice	Better Choice
Creamy Soup (Ex: Cream of Broccoli)	Broth Soup (Ex: Minestrone)
Butter	Unsalted Butter
Unsalted Butter	Vegetable Oil Spray or Olive Oil
Yogurt	Fat Free Yogurt
Sauce	Plain Yogurt mixed with Dill or Cucumber
Sandwich with meat and cheese	Raw or Grilled Vegetables on Pita Bread
Vegetables on Pita Bread	Salad
White Bread	Whole Wheat Bread
Potato Chips, Pretzels or Tortilla Chips	Dill Pickles, Raw Vegetables, or Fruit
Potato Chips and Dip	Raw vegetables and hummus, raw vegetables and salsa, or raw vegetables and a dip made with fat free sour cream
Canned Vegetables	Fresh Vegetables
Lasagna or Ravioli	Spaghetti and Meat Balls
Spaghetti and Meatballs	Linguine with Shrimp
Macaroni and Cheese	Pasta with olive oil, garlic, and chopped tomatoes
Regular Pasta	Whole Wheat Pasta
Veal Parmesan	Chicken Parmesan
Thick Crust Pizza	Thin Crust Pizza
Alfredo Sauce	Marinara Sauce
Enchilada	Shrimp Taco
Chicken Taco	Chicken Taco Salad
Beans and Rice	Beans
Hot Dog	Grilled Chicken Sandwich

151

Choice	Better Choice
Cheeseburger	Hamburger
Hamburger	Turkey Burger
Grilled Cheese Sandwich	Turkey Sandwich
Breaded Fish or Fish Sticks	Grilled or Broiled Fish
Egg Roll	Spring Roll
Shrimp Tempura	Shrimp Chop Suey
Soy Sauce	Low Sodium Soy Sauce (green top)
White Rice	Brown Rice
Cream Pie	Fruit Pie
Fruit Pie	Fresh Fruit
Ice Cream	Fat Free Frozen Yogurt
Cookies	Fat Free Sugar Free Pudding
Hot Dog	Bowl of Chili
Foot Long Sub Sandwich	Six Inch Sub Sandwich (no mayo)
French Fries	Baked Sweet Potato Fries
Mayonnaise	Ketchup or Mustard
Mashed Potatoes	Baked Potato, no toppings
Baked Potato	Whipped Cauliflower
Hashed Browned Potatoes	Fresh Fruit or Tomato Slices
Cheese Platter	Vegetable Platter
Cream Cheese	Reduced Fat Cream Cheese
Cheese	Tomato or Mushrooms
Salt	Pepper
Frozen Foods	Fresh Foods
Canned Vegetables	Fresh Vegetables
Dinner Sized Plate	Salad Sized Plate
Any Item, Large	Any Item, Small

Nutritional Labeling

Nutrition Facts are listed on packaged goods. They are a wealth of information and help you to make good food choices. Take the time when you are shopping at the grocery store and look at the Nutrition Facts and compare products before you purchase them. Just noticing how much fat and/or calories are in a particular product might help you to pick an alternative that has less calories and fat.

Also note the serving size on the Nutrition Facts. One bag of chips might seem to have not many calories until you find how many servings are supposed to be in that bag. The same is true for packaged cookies. Even the sugar free cookies pack on the pounds when you devour more than two at a time.

Nutrition Facts

Serving Size 3 oz. (85g)

Amount Per Serving	As Served
Calories 38	**Calories from Fat** 0

	% Daily Value
Total Fat 0g	0%
Saturated Fat 0g	0%
Cholesterol 0g	0%
Sodium 0g	2%
Total Carbohydrate 0g	3%
Dietary Fiber 0g	8%
Sugars 0g	
Protein 0g	

Vitamin A 270%	•	Vitamin C 10%
Calcium 2%	•	Iron 0%

Percent Daily Values are based on a 2,000 calorie diet. Your daily values may be higher or lower depending on your calorie needs:

	Calories	2,000	2,500
Total Fat	Less than	65g	80g
Sat Fat	Less than	20g	80g
Cholesterol	Less than	300mg	300mg
Sodium	Less than	2,400mg	2,400mg
Total Carbohydrate		300g	375g
Dietary Fiber		25g	30g

About the Author

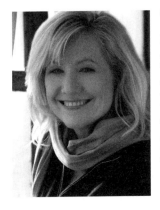

The author, Karen Batenic, is a single mother of three daughters with 25 years of business experience. She is a former Vice President of Human Resources and Executive Coach, consistently advising and counseling people at all levels in the organization. Karen has done public speaking on a regular basis to business audiences throughout the United States and has experience as a guest co-host for a Chicago TV show on health-related women's issues.

After years of starting every Monday morning on a new diet, she won her War on Weight and has lost dozens of pounds, without exercising, by Letting Go.

Notes

Notes